a guide to
back pain

Katherine Wright

Published 2010 by Geddes and Grosset,
144 Port Dundas Road, Glasgow, G4 0HZ, Scotland

© Geddes and Grosset 2010

Illustrations by Mark Mechan

ISBN 978 1 84205 653 0

Printed and bound in the UK

The material contained in this book is set out in good faith for general guidance only. Whilst every effort has been made to ensure that the information in this book is accurate, relevant and up to date, this book is sold on the condition that neither the author nor the publisher can be found legally responsible for the consequences of any errors or omissions.

Diagnosis and treatment are skilled undertakings which must always be carried out by a doctor and not from the pages of a book.

Contents

1. Introduction

Back pain is a universal human experience, being an ailment that affects most people in one form or another at some stage in life. The historical record, in addition to literature from different parts of the world, contains many references to back pain and while archaeological evidence is much harder to come by, there are certain tantalizing indicators that suggest the affliction would not have been unknown to our earliest human ancestors. Indeed, some experts suggest that the experience of back pain is linked to the fact that in evolutionary terms, the human body has had too short a time to adapt to being upright and bipedal, having originally descended from an ancestor that walked on all-fours! Whatever the truth of this, there is no doubt that the vertical state subjects the human body to a unique set of functional and 'engineering' challenges. The brunt of these forces are borne by the 'rod' that maintains the body's upright stance, in other words, the whole complex of structures that make up the human back. When there is some form of dysfunction in one or more components of this complex, the conditions are ripe for back pain to strike.

The aim of this book is to provide straightforward, useful information about the workings of the human back and the things that may go wrong to cause pain. Also, to explore the complete experience of back pain from many different angles, some of which may, at first sight, seem surprising. An example is the usefulness of analysing one's own personal attitudes, beliefs and possible misconceptions with regard to this condition. Finally, it is hoped that the book will provide guidance on the alleviation and management of back pain, from self-help measures to medical approaches and from complementary therapies to lifestyle factors. A broadbrush approach is particularly appropriate in relation to back pain as it is a problem that has many ramifications, not only for the individual sufferer but also for friends and family, the work place, economy and society as a whole.

However, this guide should not be used as a substitute for obtaining sound medical advice, especially in the event of severe and prolonged pain or if other symptoms are also present. As with all conditions and illnesses, if you are worried about your back pain you should always seek advice and reassurance, either from your own general practitioner (GP) or from a reputable substitute such as NHS Direct:

NHS Direct Helpline 0845 4647
www.nhsdirect.nhs.uk

2. Back Pain Statistics

As already stated, back pain can be regarded as an almost universal human experience. It has been estimated that 8 out of 10 people will suffer from it at some point in their lifetime and, perhaps surprisingly, back pain is as common among adolescent children as it is in adults. In Western countries, in any given year, between 15 and 49% of adults will experience at least one episode of back pain. A survey of results for the UK in the year 2003, revealed that 49% of adults reported suffering from back pain that had persisted for at least 24 hours. The peak age range at which back pain is most prevalent spans the middle years of adult life, between 35 to 55 years of age.

In over 90% of all cases, the episode is one of *acute simple back pain* (*see* page 21) and the person recovers completely within 4–6 weeks. However, even a single event increases the risk of recurrence. In up to 7% of people, the problem persists to become *chronic*. A diagnosis of *chronic back pain* is applicable when the pain has been constantly present for 3 months or longer.

In the UK, 40% of people with back pain seek help from their GP and 10% choose to consult a specialist in complementary medicine, particularly an *osteopath, chiropractor* or *acupuncturist*. The cost to the National Health Service of the treatment and management of back pain is in excess of one billion pounds each year. Of this total, more than £500 million is spent on hospital-based care, £140 million on GP consultations and £150 million on physiotherapy treatments delivered by the NHS. Additionally, approximately £565 million of private health care costs are devoted to back pain on an annual basis. A considerable proportion of these costs (approximately 80%), relate to the treatment of those with chronic back pain in whom the overall impact is high. These people frequently experience a reduction in their quality of life since chronic back pain often has adverse effects upon employment and leisure activities and on family and social relationships.

The economic impact of back pain is considerable. In the year 2003–4, 1% of the working population was absent from the work place on any one day due to back pain, equivalent to the loss of 5 million working days. Back pain is the most common reason for prolonged sickness leave among manual workers and the second most prevalent among those in other occupations. All in all, it has been estimated that these losses account for 1–2% of GDP in Western countries. Not surprisingly, these factors ensure that back pain features quite highly on the agendas of most national governments.

3. The Nature of Pain

Before beginning to look at back pain itself, it is useful to first explore the nature of pain in a more general way. The International Association for the Study of Pain (IASP), defines pain as follows: 'An unpleasant sensory and emotional experience associated with actual or potential tissue damage or described in terms of such damage.' The complicated nature of pain is neatly encompassed within this definition. It reveals that pain is not just a matter of an automatic response to a hurt but involves the mind and emotions – all those psychological factors that are mediated by the brain and are unique to each individual. These factors often have a considerable part to play in the manner in which back pain is experienced.

The type of pain that is most easily understood is termed *sudden onset* or, more commonly, *acute*. Acute pain is something that everyone experiences from time to time, whether the cause is relatively minor – perhaps a cut, bump, fall, sting or bite – or something more serious such as a fractured bone. The pain in this case may vary in intensity but it instantly alerts the individual to the fact that something untoward has occurred, usually involving some degree of tissue damage. It serves as a warning to stop and take action, both to nurture the hurt and to avoid the risk of incurring further harm. Acute pain serves a useful purpose, both for the person concerned in the incident and in a wider, evolutionary sense. It hopefully ensures that the individual survives the experience and is able to appreciate its value. Acute pain may have evolved, and persists, as a survival tactic for our species and it works at its best when it acts as a warning to prevent damage from being sustained in our day-to-day encounters with potentially harmful elements in the environment. Examples might include withdrawal of a hand that has strayed too close to a fire or stepping back, when barefoot, if something sharp has been trodden on.

Of course, in many instances of acute pain, tissue damage is sustained as a result of some accidental event. In this case, the sensory receptors in the affected part are stimulated and electrical impulses are sent to the brain where they are evaluated and interpreted as pain and damage. The term *nociceptive pain* is sometimes used to describe pain associated with tissue injury. In all these situations, the pain usually subsides and eventually disappears as healing takes place and this generally happens over a fairly limited time period.

A more complicated type of pain to consider is termed *persistent* or, more usually, *chronic*. A person is said to be suffering from *chronic pain* when the pain has been present for 12 weeks (3 months) or longer. The most significant difference between these two types is that chronic pain does not act as any form of warning signal. In some cases, especially if a known, ongoing problem is present, such as a condition affecting an organ or a degenerative disorder of the musculo-skeletal system, a cause can be diagnosed and action can be taken to relieve the situation. Chronic pain can have its origin in discernible nerve damage or abnormal nerve function in which case, the cause is termed to be *neuropathic*. Examples include foot problems in diabetes and 'phantom limb' pain, where an amputee continues to feel persistent, painful sensations coming from a limb that has been surgically removed. However, in other cases of chronic pain it is recognized that the cause does not lie with any actual nerve or tissue damage. One theory is that, for reasons remaining not fully understood, the central nervous system becomes sensitized and enters 'overdrive' mode so that signals that should be felt as harmless are experienced as pain. This type of *chronic pain syndrome* is quite often at work in cases of persistent back pain.

In medical and scientific circles, pain is acknowledged to be a highly complex response, the understanding of which remains the subject of considerable research and debate. Pain studies in human subjects continue to reveal that pain is even more complicated than was previously suspected and unravelling it lies at the heart of understanding the workings of the brain itself.

It has long been known that our perception and interpretation of pain is mediated within several areas of the brain, with the *cerebral cortex* being of critical importance. In the classical view of pain represented by the *convergent model*, pain is held to be closely related to the sense of touch, with neurons (nerve fibres) located in the deep *dorsal horn* of the spinal cord (a distinct part, also known as the *posterior column* where sensory signals are relayed) being particularly involved. These dorsal horn neurons are activated by sensory signals of pressure, temperature, touch and damage from all areas of the body and relay onward signals to the brain. It is believed that the signals *converge* and messages are sent to a specialized part of the cortex that deals with touch – the *somato-sensory cortex*. This is believed to form the heart of a widely distributed *neuromatrix* that is able to distinguish pain from other sensations. The convergent model is able to explain certain types of pain, such as *referred pain* (pain that has its origin in a deep structure but is felt to be coming from another distant area), *allodynia* (in which a person feels pain in response to a non-painful stimulus such as a light touch), and *hyperalgesia* (a greatly increased sensitivity to pain which may be felt in discrete areas or more widely from all over the body), in terms of sensitization and 'crossed wires'. It is thought that in these cases not only are inappropriate signals being sent but also there is misinterpretation in those areas of the brain responsible for processing them. The convergent model appears to provide answers but also has its shortcomings, one of the most apparent being the inability to adequately explain why human beings experience different pain sensations – pricking, stabbing, burning, gnawing, aching and so on.

Some recent research has provided evidence that painful stimuli may in fact travel along their own special pathways to the brain. The neurons believed to be involved are called *lamina 1 neurons* and they occur in the superficial layer of the dorsal horn of the spinal cord. It is thought that particular, specialized groups of lamina 1 neurons may be able to distinguish the different types of pain and are activated in response to specific stimuli. Additional scientific evidence may point to the existence of *pain centres* in the brain, with a region called the *parieto-insular cortex* or *interoceptive cortex* being crucially important. The interoceptive cortex has only been found to occur in primates and is especially highly developed in human beings. Another area lying within the frontal cortex, called the *anterior cingulate,* is activated when pain is being experienced along with other regions that include the *cerebellum, amygdala* and *striatum.* Some researchers believe that the anterior cingulate is critically involved in the emotional aspects of pain. Hence, in this alternative *homeostatic model* of pain, it is proposed that there is a physical component centred on the parieto-insular cortex and an emotional element centred on the anterior cingulate. In this model, it is believed that the perception of pain evolved in primates as an extension of the mechanisms that alert the brain to the internal, physiological state of the body (*homeostasis*).

Both models offer insights into the workings of the brain in relation to pain but there are many questions that remain. One of the most important is the influence of the mind on the actual experience of pain – that whole complex of interaction between intangible beliefs and emotions and the physical entity that is pain. The umbrella term *psychosocial factors* deals with the influence of the mind and emotions upon our individual experience of pain and it is wide-ranging, including as it does anxiety, stress, depression, familial and social isolation and the many aspects of life that have a bearing upon these. Psychosocial factors have a considerable bearing on pain and are particularly influential with regard to chronic pain, both in its development and as a barrier to recovery.

One final factor to be considered is the concept of the *pain threshold*, defined as the degree or extent of stimulation that needs to be applied before pain is felt. A discovery made within the last few years may help to explain the variation seen among people in their ability to withstand pain. The answer may partly lie with a gene that exists in two forms or variants known as *val* and *met*. Both are involved in the manufacture of an enzyme called *catechol-O-methyl-transferase* (COMT) that is responsible for breaking down *neurotransmitters* (chemicals that allow messages to be sent) such as *dopamine*. However, there are slight differences in the efficacy of the COMT produced, with the val gene generating a more potent version of the enzyme. It is believed that an accumulation of biochemicals, such as dopamine, restricts the brain's ability to produce its own natural painkillers, the *endorphins* (endogenous opioids). Individuals inherit one copy of the gene from each parent so some possess two val, others two met and the remainder, one of each. Some studies have suggested that those with two val genes possess a greater ability to remove dopamine and experience less pain than those with two met genes. Critically, those who are 'two met' also reported fewer negative emotions connected with pain. People with one copy of each gene showed varying responses lying somewhere between the two extremes. While this may seem to be a matter mainly of scientific interest, it should perhaps have a broader application in challenging attitudes. This is because, all too often, someone complaining of a pain that is not considered by others to be significant or bad enough to merit sympathy is treated with a dismissive or negative response. Such attitudes are sometimes encountered by those suffering from back pain and usually have a negative effect upon the person's morale and are certainly not helpful.

4. What is Back Pain and What is Its Cause?

The answers to these questions are perhaps not as obvious as they may first seem. When asked about back pain, most people think of the lower and possibly the middle areas of their back and will probably point to these regions when questioned. But they do not automatically include the legs or the neck and shoulders, or realize that a dysfunction in one part of the spine can result in pain in an area somewhat remote from the origin of the problem.

Also, on first consideration, the majority of people think of back pain as being the primary entity in itself whereas, in fact, it is always a *symptom* of an underlying problem. So a broad answer might be that back pain can be defined as pain that owes its origin in some way to disorder, dysfunction or damage to one or more of the complex of structures that make up the spine (vertebral column). But the nature of the pain and the way it operates and is perceived is often far more complex than this answer implies.

Back structures comprise:

- *Vertebrae* (bones)
- *Intervertebral discs* (cushioning pads located between vertebrae)
- *Ligaments* (strong, fibrous bands of connective tissue that join bones together)
- *Spinal cord* (the vitally important nerve bundle that carries electrical signals to and from the brain to the rest of the body)
- *Spinal nerves* (paired segmental nerves that lead off from the spinal cord on either side at the level of each vertebra)
- *Muscles* (large and small that connect to the spine and allow movements to occur)
- *Tendons* (tough, inelastic 'ropes', varying in length and thickness, that join muscles to bones).

Of all of these, it is the vertebrae that comprise the basic building blocks of the back, consisting of 34 bones or segments. The lowest 10 of these are mostly fused together so that often, the spine is described as comprising 24 vertebrae, each stacked one on top of the other from the 'tail bone' to the neck. The back can be thought of as structural complex that is a miracle of engineering, expected to perform a multitude of tasks, some of them conflicting, day-in-day-out over the course of a lifetime! It is perhaps hardly surprising that things may go wrong and that when this happens, pain may result.

As to what goes wrong, back pain arises for four main reasons:

- *Injury* to one or more structures of the back
- *Degeneration*, usually age-related changes to back structures. Degenerative changes affecting the structure of the spine occur almost universally and inevitably as a result of aging and these are often collectively referred to as 'wear and tear'.
- *Congenital* abnormalities affecting back structures, present at birth but not necessarily causing immediate problems
- *Illnesses* or *conditions* arising during the course of a lifetime but that are not congenital.

Quite often, it is a combination of these that is ultimately responsible for back pain but there may be other factors at work contributing to the way the pain is experienced.

From looking at the above list of reasons, it could appear at first sight that back pain should be a relatively straightforward condition to understand – a simple matter of cause and effect. It might seem that once the cause has been identified, it should then be possible to correct or eliminate it and that the effect of this would be for the pain to disappear. Unfortunately, the situation in many cases is rather more complicated. Hence, in modern medicine, a somewhat different approach is taken to classify back pain – one in which 'cause' is perhaps given a lower degree of importance.

During the early 1990s, the UK government, concerned at the prevalence of back pain among the population and its human and economic consequences, appointed an advisory committee to examine the issues and devise strategies on how best to tackle the problem. One of the recommendations was to suggest the adoption of a *triage* approach to the classification of patients presenting with back pain – a concept that is more usually associated with large-scale emergencies and hospital casualty departments. *Back pain triage* assigns sufferers to one of three initial categories at the stage of a first consultation with the GP or health-care provider and this system is the one that is now in general use. These categories are *simple back pain*, *nerve root pain* or *radicular pain* and *other pathology* as described below.

Back pain triage

Simple back pain
It may be surprising to discover that about 94% of sufferers fall into this category and that for around 70% of their number, no concrete and definitive cause for their symptoms is ever found. Most people in this group experience the pain in their lower back (*lumbar* region) and, if nerves are irritated, it may also be felt (usually one-sidedly) in the buttocks and thighs. In the vast majority of cases (9 out of every 10 people who have an acute attack), the symptoms greatly improve within 2 weeks and subside and disappear completely after 4–6 weeks. However, there may be a recurrence at some future time.

Some people, especially if their symptoms are severe, may feel that a diagnosis of simple back pain implies some sort of slur, as though they are not being taken seriously when reporting a high degree of pain. But it must be remembered that the term is not intended to reflect upon the severity of the pain in any way. It is well recognized that pain in this instance can vary from extremely severe and disabling, especially at the onset of an attack, to moderate or relatively mild. However, if the pain is intense at first, it generally subsides to a more bearable level within 2 days and it also tends to vary in its intensity depending upon movement and activity. If anything, the term 'simple back pain' reflects the prevalence of the problem and also, that it usually arises from an interaction of disorders and dysfunctions in several components of the back that are too complex to unravel. Further, that even if it were possible to work out exactly what is happening, the pain in most cases, will have subsided or disappeared completely before any investigation had been completed.

It is arguable as to whether a different label reflecting this complexity might have been more useful, if only because some people may find it hard to accept that they are suffering from simple back pain. This is important since failure to accept and fully grasp the implications of the diagnosis, particularly any reluctance to believe that the symptoms will subside and improve, may be a barrier to recovery and increase the risk of development of chronic back pain. Again, for anyone receiving this diagnosis, it is important to realize that tests and scans are considered inappropriate because these will not reveal anything useful about the condition. The advice that you will almost certainly be given is that even if you must rest to begin with, you should start to move about as early as you can and resume normal activities as soon as possible. You will probably be advised to take over-the-counter analgesic preparations in the first instance and only if the pain is extremely severe are you likely to be prescribed any other form of medication.

Nerve root pain or radicular pain

Nerve root pain is relatively uncommon, affecting about 5% of those with back pain. The direct cause is pressure, pinching or irritation of one of the *segmental spinal nerves* leading off from the spinal cord, sometimes alternatively described as a *trapped nerve*. The area most usually affected is the lower back but it can also occur in the neck, in which case pain is often additionally felt in the shoulder and arm. Pain is experienced along the length of the nerve and, in the case of the lower back, may extend to the buttock and down through the thigh and calf as far as the foot on the affected side. The best-known and commonest example involves the *sciatic nerve,* which is relatively susceptible to pressure and results in the condition known as *sciatica*.

Nerve root pain varies in severity but at its worst is intense and highly demoralizing. In addition to pain, there may be numbness, tingling, muscular weakness in the leg and 'pins-and-needles' sensations. The pain is often relieved by lying still, especially at the start of the attack and is made worse by any movements using the back and by sneezing or coughing. The cause of the compression in most cases is a *prolapsed disc*, although in elderly persons, it is more likely to be *spinal stenosis* (*see* page 89). When pain is intense, it is not always possible for the sufferer to obtain relief, whatever the position adopted, and the person is likely to lose sleep and may be unable to eat properly. This soon leads to feelings of depression and debility and in these instances it is necessary to ask for medical advice, as should also be the case if numbness and muscular weakness are experienced. There are a number of preparations available on prescription that work in various ways to ease pain, relieve muscle tension and act directly upon nerves. The patient may also benefit from onward referral to specialist orthopaedic or musculo-skeletal services or to a pain clinic.

In those less severely affected, the advice given is likely to be essentially similar to that for simple back pain. It is best try and avoid complete bed-rest but, if this is necessary, it should be for no more than 2 days. Gentle activity is recommended and sitting in one position for any length of time should be avoided. When sitting, a firm chair offering good back support should be used rather than a soft armchair. Normal activities should be resumed as soon as possible but need to be undertaken in a measured way, so that tasks are broken up into short phases of work interspersed with rest. If symptoms do not respond to these measures or if they start to get worse, or if sleep is continually being interrupted by pain, medical advice should be sought and prescription medication is likely to be needed.

Other pathology

Less than 1% of people with back pain have a serious, underlying disease or condition that is causing their symptoms. Within this group it is more likely, although by no means exclusively so, for the pain to start gradually and grow steadily worse over time. Also, there is often a far weaker relationship between the amount of activity undertaken and the severity of the pain. Patients in this category will almost certainly seek medical help at some point and in the first instance the doctor may, or may not have reason to suspect that an underlying condition is present. However, if there are any grounds for suspicion, further investigations will begin immediately and these may include a physical examination, blood tests, x-rays, a computerized topography (CT) scan and a magnetic resonance imaging (MRI) scan.

Rare causes include malignancy, possibly of the spine, bones, bladder, pancreas or kidney, viral infections, such as shingles and meningitis and prostatitis (in men), fibromyalgia and kidney disorders. Also, there are various congenital disorders of the spine and other unusual causes that may include back pain among a spectrum of symptoms such as Crohn's disease and ulcerative colitis. But a far more likely cause of back pain in this category is one of the various forms of arthritis – not only spinal arthritis but also other types that may affect the spine as well as other bones and joints. Osteoporosis poses a particular risk of damage to spinal structures, particularly in older women. (*See also* individual entries from page 75.)

5. The Structures of the Back

In order to understand back pain, it is useful to first look at the structures of the back in somewhat greater detail, beginning with the spine and its constituent vertebrae.

The spine and its constituent vertebrae

As noted already, the spine or vertebral column is made up of 34 bones, of which the lowest 10 have mostly lost their individual identity by being fused together. In adults, the spine is about 70 cm (28 ins) in length and, surprisingly, there is little variation between individuals, with differences in height being governed primarily by the length of the legs. The spinal column performs many useful functions and these include providing structural support and balance; forming the connection between the trunk of the body and the lower limbs; providing anchorage for muscles, ligaments and tendons, and protection for vital organs and especially the spinal cord; enabling a wide range of movements to take place, such as forwards, backwards and sideways bending and rotation, and contributing to the movements of the limbs.

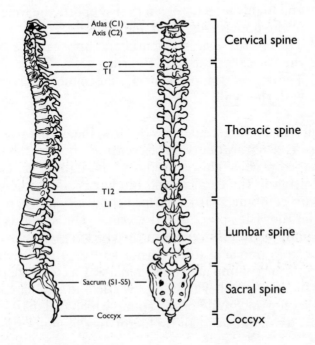

Atlas (C1)
Axis (C2)
C7
T1
T12
L1
Sacrum (S1–S5)
Coccyx

Cervical spine

Thoracic spine

Lumbar spine

Sacral spine

Coccyx

Fig 1 The 5 regions of the spine

The spine is divided into 5 regions (*see* Fig 1) and these comprise, in ascending order:

1. The *coccyx* or tail bone, consisting of 3 to 5 mainly fused small bones that nonetheless retain some slight flexibility.
2. The *sacral spine*, comprising 5 fused vertebrae that make up the triangular-shaped *sacrum*.

3. The *lumbar spine* of the lower back, a strong, robust and highly mobile region that supports the weight of the upper body, head and arms.
4. The *thoracic spine* in the mid and upper regions of the back that supports the ribcage.
5. The *cervical spine* of the neck that connects directly with the skull.

Figure 1, showing a side view of the spine, illustrates that there is a natural curvature creating an open, shallow, s-shaped profile. This is produced by slight concavity or hollowing in the cervical and lumbar regions, known as *lordosis*, combined with a natural convexity in the region of the thoracic spine, called *kyphosis*. The shape is produced by slight differences in the thickness of the vertebrae from one side to the other so that the individual units of the column are stacked in a way as to make them a little offset, rather than in a vertical line. Changes in the 'sweep' or profile of the spine, which can arise from a variety of causes, can be factor in the generation of pain.

1. The coccyx

The coccyx or tail bone is the lowest part of the spine and consists of 3 to 5 fused and reduced vertebrae, with 4 being the usual number. The coccyx is a vestigial tail surrounded by muscle and located beneath the sacrum. Although it is held in place quite firmly by surrounding tissues, it does retain a degree of flexibility. It can be generally associated with lower back pain or be the focus in itself, either as a result of trauma and injury, such as displacement or fracture, or due to a condition known as *coccydinia* (*see* page 96).

2. The sacrum

The sacrum consists of 5 fused vertebrae, producing a roughly triangular-shaped bone that forms the back wall of the *pelvic* or *hip girdle*. The individual elements of the sacrum are designated, in abbreviated form, S1 to S5. The sacrum joins at either side with the paired *ilia* and the joints so formed are called the *sacroiliac joints*. Each ilium is a large ear-shaped bone and it is fused with two other bones (the *pubis* and *ischium*) to form the hip complex on either side. The upper part of the sacrum provides a sloping surface to which the lowest of the lumbar vertebrae is firmly secured. The sacrum itself is bound into place by some of the thickest and strongest ligaments in the body. Despite this, the sacroiliac joint is capable of a minute degree of movement although its main function is one of strength in supporting the upper body.

3. The lumbar spine

The 5 lumbar vertebrae are designated, in abbreviated form, L1 to L5 (*see* Fig 1). They are the stoutest and strongest of all the individual units of the spine, gradually decreasing in size in ascending order from L5 to L1. Lumbar vertebrae are slightly thicker or wedged at the front, producing a gentle forward curve and a natural hollow at the back, the lumbar *lordosis*.

The structure of a free spinal vertebra: Lumbar vertebrae are built to bear weight but all the free vertebrae of the spine have the same basic structure. The main part of each vertebra, known as the *vertebral body*, can be seen to be slightly narrower towards the centre in side-view (Fig 2a), giving the appearance of a 'waist'. This arrangement helps to spread the load but the main strength comes from the internal structure of the vertebra, comprising a three-dimensional 'scaffolding' of upright columns and horizontal bars.

Behind the body of each vertebra towards the outside, the bone continues as a ring with a central hole or *foramen* and various bony protuberances. Paired bony knobs protrude from the uppermost surface of the ring of bone on either side of the foramen and these are known as the *superior articular processes*. Likewise at the bottom, another pair arise known as the *inferior articular processes*. It is at the tips of these that two adjacent vertebrae above and below make bone-to-bone contact with one another. For example, the superior articular processes of L2 extend upwards and form a joint on either side with the inferior articular processes of L1, pointing downwards from immediately above. Similarly, the inferior articular processes of L2 project downwards and form a joint on either side with the upward pointing, superior articular processes of L3, positioned beneath. The small areas where these contacts are made are called *zygapophysial,* apophyseal or, more commonly, *facet joints* (Fig 2c).

Like many of those in the body, facet joints are of a type known as *synovial* or moveable joints, each of which has four elements and these are: the two bones themselves; a layer of *cartilage* covering the ends of the bones, making them smooth; a sheath of fibrous tissue, called

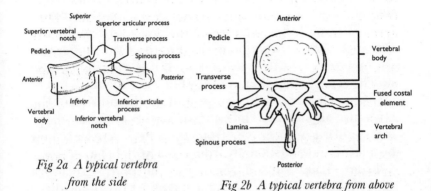

Fig 2a A typical vertebra
from the side

Fig 2b A typical vertebra from above

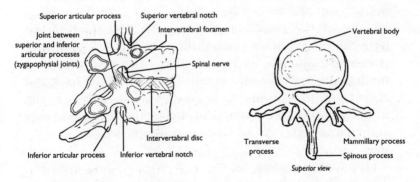

Fig 2c Intervertebral foramina

Fig 2d A lumbar vertebra

the *capsule*, from which ligaments form that bind the joints together; the *synovial membrane* or *synovium*, the inner lining of the capsule, which secretes a thick fluid called *synovia* to lubricate the joint. They allow for a degree of free movement between individual vertebrae and since the angles vary throughout the length of the spine, this arrangement confers flexibility. But facet joints also notch securely together, thereby blocking shearing forces while muscles and ligaments maintain the tension of the structure as a whole. The joints are richly innervated, being supplied with nerves from the nerve roots at their own level and additionally from one level above.

From either side of the bony ring of the vertebra (known as the *neural arch)* a pair of short protuberances project called *transverse processes* and lastly, from the hindmost part, a single *spinous process* points outwards horizontally (Fig 2d). The ends of the spinous processes are the knobs that can be seen and felt externally when looking at the back and they occupy a central groove between muscle masses on either side. The function of transverse and spinous processes is to provide attachment points for the many smaller muscles of the back and these run in various directions. Contractions of the muscles pull on the levers provided by the bony processes and enable vertebrae to move in different ways.

4. The thoracic spine

The thoracic spine, which extends from the base of the neck to just above the waist, is the longest part of the back and has the profile of a gentle outward curve, making the central sweep of the s-shape. It comprises 12 vertebrae, designated T1 to T12 and these are finer and less robust than those of the lumbar spine. They gradually increase in size downwards, from T1 to T12 (*see* Fig 1).

Both the transverse and spinous processes are longer and thinner in the thoracic region than those of the lumbar region and a further difference is that the spinous processes project downwards rather than horizontally. Each thoracic vertebra has a relatively large *intervertebral*

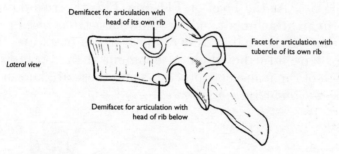

Lateral view

Demifacet for articulation with head of its own rib

Facet for articulation with tubercle of its own rib

Demifacet for articulation with head of rib below

Fig 3a A thoracic vertebra from the side

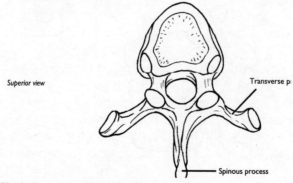

Superior view

Transverse p

Spinous process

Fig 3b A thoracic vertebra from above

foramen to accommodate the nerve roots that arise from the spinal cord. The effect of this is that nerve root compression is less likely to arise in this part of the spine.

An important function of the thoracic spine is to provide attachment points for 12 pairs of ribs. These sweep round in a curve from the *sternum* (breastbone) at the front of the chest and attach at either side at the level of the junction between the thoracic vertebrae. The rib-vertebra junctions are called *costovertebral joints* or *facets* (Fig 3c). At the level of T11 and T12, the ribs do not form an attachment and are known as *floating ribs*. In addition to the main costovertebral joints or facets, the ribs have a further slight attachment at the very top of each of the transverse processes and these are known as the *costotransverse joints* or *facets*.

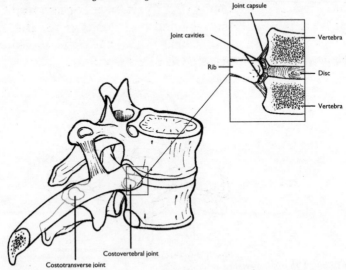

Fig 3c Costovertebral joints

The net effect of the anchorage of the ribs is to reduce the mobility of the thoracic spine when compared to that of the lumbar and cervical regions and the principle function of this part of the spine is to provide stability for the ribcage and the vital organs it contains. A further important role is to provide core stability for the highly mobile neck and head that are located directly above. Although rib anchorage restricts movement, it does not prevent it altogether. Thoracic vertebrae should possess the ability to glide and, most importantly, to rotate and problems can arise if one or more costo-vertebral junctions are too tight, thereby tethering the vertebrae and leading to stiffness and pain.

5. The cervical spine

The cervical spine comprises 7 vertebrae, designated C1 to C7. It is further sub-divided into two regions; the upper cervical spine comprising C1 and C2 and the lower cervical spine comprising C3 to C7 (*see* Fig 1).

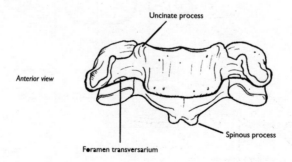

Fig 4a A cervical vertebra from the side

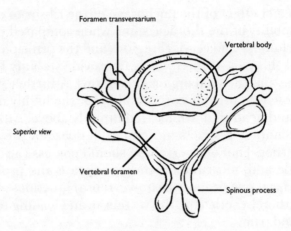

Foramen transversarium

Vertebral body

Superior view

Vertebral foramen

Spinous process

Fig 4b A cervical vertebra from above

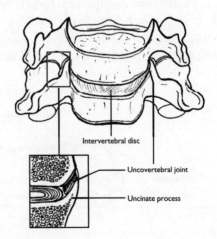

Intervertebral disc

Uncovertebral joint

Uncinate process

Fig 4c Uncovertebral joints

Cervical vertebrae are the most delicate of all those present in the spine. Each has a round vertebral body with a triangular-shaped vertebral foramen and pair of transverse processes projecting from each side, each containing a *foramen transversarium*, and a flattish spinous process protruding horizontally.

In addition to facet joints, additional bone-to-bone contacts occur between cervical vertebrae. The body of each is slightly ridged at either side (*uncinate process*) and it makes contact with the vertebra above by means of specialized joints of Lushka or *uncovertebral joints*. These joints provide additional bony protection for the *intervertebral discs* and this means that prolapsed discs rarely occur in this region (*see* Fig 4c opposite).

C1 and C2 of the upper cervical spine are uniquely modified and specialized vertebrae (*see* Figs 4d and 4e on page 38). C1, known as the *atlas*, consists of a ring of bone that is thickened into two masses on each side and joined by an *anterior* and *posterior arch*. The atlas forms direct contact with a flattened bone at the base of the skull called the *occiput* or *occipital bone*. Two rounded projections, known as *condyles*, protrude from the occipital bone on each side and these fit neatly into two corresponding scooped-out hollows on either side of the atlas. It is these joints that allow for the nodding action of the head. C2, known as the *axis*, is likewise specialized but in a different way. It has a long, tooth-like peg of bone, called the *dens* or *odontoid peg*, that projects vertically through a central hole in the overlying atlas. The collar and pivot effect produced enables the head and the atlas to swivel and rotate upon the axis and the lower spine.

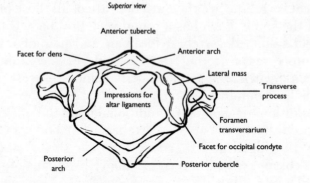

Fig 4d Atlas cervical vertebra

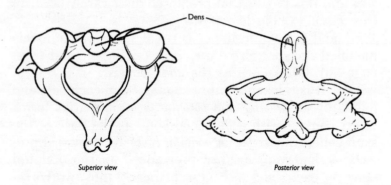

Fig 4e Axis cervical vertebra

The neck is richly supplied with an array of muscles that control all the interplay of movement of which this region is capable. Due to the high degree of movement, smooth running of the facet joints is critical to the correct operation of the region. Equally, disharmony or blockage of facet joint movement, usually caused in some way by muscular tension or strain, can easily result in inflammation and rigidity and be a major contributor to painful conditions of the neck.

Intervertebral discs

Intervertebral discs are found between all the vertebrae in the spinal column other than those that are fused and are located between the body of each individual segment. Discs resemble tough yet compressible cushions and are often described as acting like shock absorbers and ball bearings combined. They are at their thickest between lumbar vertebrae, protecting the bones while at the same time endowing this region with much of its freedom of movement.

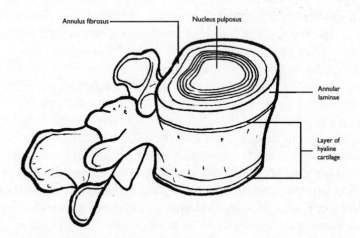

Fig 5 Structure of an intervertebral disc

39

Each disc has two parts – the outer layer known as the *annular fibrosus* and an inner central nucleus called the *nucleus pulposus*. The annular fibrosus has an outer ring of collagen surrounding layers of fibrous cartilage that can be likened to a car tyre, with a criss-cross pattern of diagonal fibres occurring in successive layers (known as *annular rings* or *annular laminae*) that confer both strength and flexibility. The nucleus pulposus is comprised of a water-based gel that can be compressed and is capable of altering its shape (*see* Fig 5).

Each intervertebral disc is lightly supplied with nerves via the segmental nerves and *dorsal root ganglions* at each level. Outward squirting of the nucleus pulposus exerts pressure on the outer, fibrous ring while at the same time absorbing and distributing the forces to which it is subjected. The net effect is to allow for a rocker-like movement between adjacent vertebrae. Fluid is absorbed into the disc from specialized layers of *hyaline cartilage* called *end plates* that line the top and bottom of each vertebral body. The fluid is absorbed through the outer layers of the disc and finds its way into the nucleus. The nucleus possesses the ability to attract and retain liquid but during all upright movement and activity, compressive forces result in a net loss of liquid. This has the effect of causing a daily reduction in disc thickness of about 10%. Fluid and nutrients are replenished during night-time sleep by means of a process called *intradiscal fluid exchange*. It is further believed that gentle, rhythmical exercise may aid rehydration.

The joints between discs and vertebral bodies are the main junctions between the stack of segments that comprise the spinal column. These joints are of a type known as *cartilaginous joints*. Characteristically, these joints are only slightly moveable at an individual level but, as has been seen, the spine possesses the remarkable ability to achieve considerable flexure over its length as a whole. The role of the joints between discs and vertebrae is to contribute to this overall degree of movement.

One final and highly significant fact regarding discs is that they undergo an inevitable degenerative change with aging. In youth the discs are well hydrated, plump and flexible but during aging, the tendency is for them to dry out and hence lose much of their substance, thickness and flexibility so that in old age, they become almost entirely fibrous in nature. The nature of this process helps to explain why *discogenic pain* is most common in the middle years of adult life, between the ages of 35 to 55 years.

The spinal cord

The spinal cord is a direct extension of the *medulla oblongata*, the lowest portion of the brain stem that leaves the skull through a large opening called the *foramen magnum*. The spinal cord then continues its downward progress through the *spinal canal*, a hollow tube surrounded by bone that is formed from the *neural rings* or *arches* of the vertebrae. The spinal cord has a slightly flattened, cylindrical shape and it is about as thick as a fountain pen. At about the level of the 2nd lumbar vertebra, it becomes much thinner and continues as a 'string' known as the *filum terminale* which ends at the coccyx.

The spinal cord is somewhat thickened in two places, in the lower cervical region and at the base of the thoracic spine, and it is from these areas that the nerves supplying the arms and legs arise. Like the brain, the spinal cord contains both *grey* and *white matter*. The grey matter exists as an H-shaped core within the surrounding white matter, with *anterior* and *posterior horns* extending through almost to the surface of the cord and giving rise to the *nerve roots*.

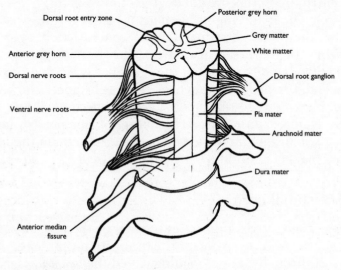

Fig 6 The spinal cord

In the centre of the H of grey matter is a hollow central canal containing *cerebral spinal fluid* that bathes and nourishes the surrounding tissue. As with the brain, the spinal cord is surrounded by three layers of membrane or *meninges* and these are composed of connective tissue. The outermost one of these is called the *dura mater* and it is tough and protective. A layer consisting of fat and blood vessels lies between this and the vertebral canal while on the inside, cerebrospinal fluid separates it from the spinal cord. The dura mater and cerebrospinal fluid also partially surround each nerve root. The innermost two membranes are called the *arachnoid mater* and *pia mater*, respectively and these are also bathed with fluid. This arrangement ensures that in all normal movements of the spine, the cord is protected and cushioned from any pressure or trauma.

Spinal nerves

Thirty-one pairs of *segmental spinal nerves* arise from the spinal cord, a pair at each segmental level on either side. Each of these arises as an *anterior* or *ventral nerve root* and a *posterior* or *dorsal nerve root* which become united before they leave the spinal canal. The combined nerve roots then leave the spinal canal through the *intervertebral foramina,* the hollow grooves in the upper and lower surfaces of the neural rings of the vertebrae. In the higher parts of the vertebral column, the spinal nerves exit almost horizontally. But lower down the angle becomes steeper so that, eventually, a fantail of nerves called the *cauda equina* (because it resembles a horse's tail) is formed. These nerves extend downwards, each finding its own particular foramen, and continue through to the sacrum and coccyx.

The *sciatic nerve* is the main nerve complex of each leg, passing down the back of the thigh and continuing into the foot. It contains nerves from several of the nerve roots issuing from the lower part of the spinal cord and it may be involved in cases of lower back pain (*see* page 87).

Within the intervertebral foramen, each dorsal nerve root widens to form the *dorsal root ganglion* which contains

43

the cell bodies of sensory nerves that feed electrical impulses back to the spinal cord. The spinal cord is a highly complex structure that not only relays information to and from the brain via the many nerves connected with it but also contains control centres of its own. It has been estimated that at the point where it enters the brain, the upper portion of the cord contains half the number of nerve fibres that are present in the lower region, with its numerous connections to the network of segmental spinal nerves.

Muscles of the spine

The spine provides an attachment for an enormous number of *muscles* and these are of a type known as *voluntary* or *striated*; voluntary because they are responsible for movement under individual control and striated due to the appearance of stripes when viewed beneath a microscope. Each muscle is enclosed in a sheath of connective tissue, called the *fascia*. Extensions of this penetrate the bulk of the muscle mass, dividing it into bundles. The bundles are composed of elongated fibres, each consisting of even finer *fibrils* and every fibre is enclosed by an elastic covering called the *sarcolemma*. Minute bundles of fine connective tissue fibres at each end of every sarcolemma are the means by which one fibre is attached to another or to connective tissue. Numerous blood capillaries supplying oxygen and nutrients run between the fibres. Additionally, each muscle fibre is supplied by a nerve fibre that penetrates the sarcolemma and then divides into many fine endings (known as an *end plate*) that spread out across the surface. By this means, contraction of the muscle is brought under the control of the central nervous system. During contraction, a muscle bunches and shortens to about two thirds of its relaxed length and blood is squeezed out as the capillaries flatten.

Back muscles form a complex arrangement and can be subdivided into two groups: *deep muscles* and *superficial muscles*. Taken together they form two columns one on each side of the spine, extending down the entire length of the back from the base of the head to the sacrum. The group that is most deep-seated comprise three layers of strong muscle that are collectively called the *transverso-spinalis muscles*.

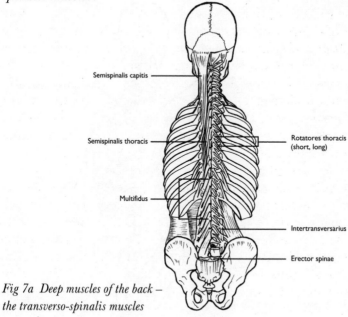

Semispinalis capitis

Semispinalis thoracis

Rotatores thoracis (short, long)

Multifidus

Intertransversarius

Erector spinae

Fig 7a Deep muscles of the back – the transverso-spinalis muscles

These are the short muscles that connect individual vertebrae, being responsible for fine movement and stability. The deepest layer of the three comprise the *rotatores,* the middle the *multifidus* and the outermost, the *semispinalis* (see Fig 7a on page 46).

Another important group, called the *erector spinae* muscles ('raisers of the spine'), overlie the transverso-spinalis and like these, they also attach only to the spine. They are large, strong muscles that extend the whole length of the back and are responsible for movement and also the provision of core stability.

The superficial muscles are the largest in the back.

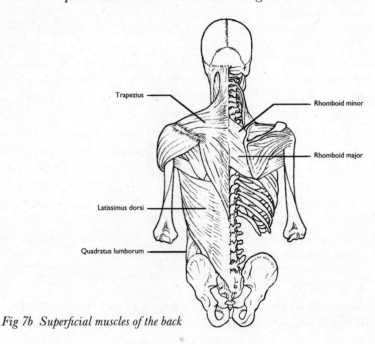

Trapezius

Rhomboid minor

Rhomboid major

Latissimus dorsi

Quadratus lumborum

Fig 7b Superficial muscles of the back

They include the *trapezius* which is responsible for shoulder movement, being attached to the cervical and thoracic spine on either side; the *latissmus dorsi*, responsible for downward and backward arm movements, being attached to the iliac crest and thoracic vertebrae; also, the *quadratus lumborium* that is attached to the iliac crest and to lumbar vertebrae and is involved in extension of the lumbar spine and sideways bending.

The *gluteus* or buttock muscles do not, strictly speaking, belong to the back – they are involved in walking and the maintenance of a standing posture – but they can be involved in lower back pain. Abdominal muscles lack the bony support provided by the ribcage and are therefore strengthened by extra sheets of fibrous tissue. They also form three layers with deeper ones, including the *transversus abdominus* and multifidus forming attachments with lumbar vertebrae. Contraction of abdominal muscles increases pressure internally, acting like a corset to support the back.

Back muscles do not work as individual entities but in groups that are in harmony with one another and thus achieve movement. They are highly sensitive and can be subject to misuse, fatigue, sprain and strain both directly and indirectly. They react to biochemical signals, such as stress hormones released into the bloodstream during emotional states such as anxiety, and are often involved during episodes of back pain.

Ligaments
Ligaments in the back provide support for the bony structures of the spine and due to their slightly elastic nature,

act to both cushion and restrain movements while at the same time allowing for a degree of 'give'. They can be divided into two main types: those that bind individual vertebrae to one another, known as *intrasegmental ligaments*; and those that run the whole length of the vertebral column, called *intersegmental ligaments*.

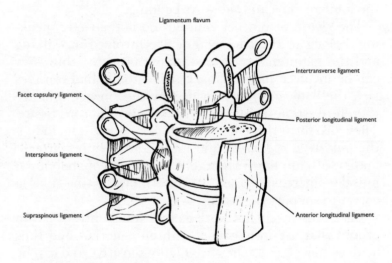

Fig 8 Ligaments of the spine

Intrasegmental ligaments include the robust *ligamentum flavum* (or yellow ligament), which connects the posterior surfaces of individual vertebrae. Also important are the *interspinous ligaments*, situated in between the spinous processes and also, the *intertransverse ligaments*, binding each transverse process on either side to the one immediately above and below in the vertebral column. A further one of note is the *supraspinous ligament* which is a thin 'rope' attached to the tip of each spinous process. The intersegmental ligaments are much longer as they provide overall support for the spine. Important among them are the *anterior* and *posterior longitudinal ligaments* that run down the front and back of all the individual vertebral bodies, respectively.

Tendons

Tendons are the tough, inelastic cords composed of *collagen* fibres that attach the muscles of the back to the bones, principally the vertebrae. A tendon concentrates the 'pull' of a muscle onto its attachment point on the bone, and the length and thickness of individual tendons can vary considerably.

A tendon may be enclosed in a tendon sheath lined with synovial membrane containing fluid (*synovia*) that reduces friction and facilitates movement.

6. The Impact of Damage or Dysfunction in One or More of the Structures of the Back

Having considered the structures of the back, it is now possible to look in a general way at how damage or dysfunction in one or more of these parts can result in pain. Given the complexity and inter-connected nature of the structures of the back, it is certainly the case that more often than not, several of them are involved when there is pain. A malfunction or injury in one part often sets up accompanying problems in the structures with which it is closely associated.

The bones of the spine, the *vertebrae*, may be a cause of pain either through injury or due to degeneration or by a combination of both these factors. Types of injury include *fractures* (of which there are three types) and these may be accompanied by *spinal dislocation*, in which one or more joints are forced out of their normal position. It is unusual for a dislocation to occur in the absence of a fracture. Degenerative disorders affecting the vertebrae include *spondylosis* or spinal arthritis and *osteoporosis* and both of these are associated with aging. Abnormal outgrowths of bone, known as *osteophytes* or *bony spurs* growing out from vertebrae may be a feature of degenerative arthritic disorders of the spine and these may be a factor in the development of *stenosis* (narrowing) of the central spinal canal or one or more of the lateral canals housing the nerve roots. A particular, progressive degenerative disorder known as *ankylosing spondylitis* affects a younger age group and may begin in childhood.

The *facet joints* between the articular processes of the vertebrae can be a cause of pain, usually resulting from a sudden awkward movement or an accidental blow or fall. The pain and 'locking' is associated with localized muscle spasm and there may be consequent inflammation within the joint and irritation of associated nerves. Wear and tear of the spine in older people, possibly accompanied by poor posture and some misalignment of the vertebrae, can subject the facet joints to undue loading pressure and result in a chronic form of pain.

The *sacroiliac joint* is a unique joint associated with the spine and its involvement in lower back pain has sometimes been controversial. However, it is now recognized that strain of this joint can cause pain, especially in the buttock on the affected side or *referred* to the groin, leg or hip. The joint may be associated with lumbar back pain and affected by inflammatory diseases such as ankylosing spondylitis.

As noted previously, *nerves* form the relay system by means of which pain messages are transmitted and interpreted so, in this sense, nerves are involved in all cases of back pain. However, more specifically, nerve root pain, in which a spinal nerve is subjected to pressure, irritation and/or inflammation, is involved in about 5% of all cases of back pain. The exact cause of the problem varies and may involve more than one of the structures adjacent to the nerve, including a protruding or prolapsed disc, muscle and/or tendon strain, ligament sprain or degenerative changes in vertebrae causing lateral canal stenosis. The central spinal canal may also become similarly narrowed (spinal stenosis) due usually but not exclusively to degenerative changes accompanying aging. This problem more commonly affects the lumbar region. In this case, direct pressure may then be exerted upon the spinal cord itself or on any of the nerves with which it is connected. The sciatic nerve is commonly involved, leading to the painful condition known as *sciatica* (see page 87). Nerve root pain can be anything from relatively mild to extremely severe with associated referred pain, numbness, pins-and-needles sensations and, in extreme cases, muscle weakness, loss of sensation and incontinence. Anyone with severe symptoms should seek medical help.

Depending upon severity, treatment may involve *prescription medication*, *spinal manipulation*, *physiotherapy*, specific *exercises* and possibly, *spinal injections* and/or *surgery*. However, it should be remembered that serious nerve root pain is rare and in most cases the more serious forms of intervention are not required. The spinal cord itself is at risk in cases of accidental trauma and injury to the back. Emergency medical aid is needed for anyone with a suspected back injury and the person should not be moved, except in cases of pressing danger, until expert help arrives. There is a need to support and stabilize the back before the patient can be moved in order to prevent damage to the spinal cord and failure to do this carries the risk of causing irreversible harm, resulting in potentially permanent disability and paralysis.

The *muscles* of the back are often implicated in pain generation. They may be the main source of pain or, perhaps more usually, become involved due to damage or strain to one of the joints of the spine. This may cause nearby muscles to become tense or strained in their turn and they may go into spasm. Acute *muscle strain*, in which there is a tear or over-stretch of a small muscle or of some of the fibres of a larger one, is nearly always the result of an accidental event, such as a blow or fall, a twisting movement or inappropriate lifting of a heavy weight. A sports injury is a common cause. The person may feel the muscle 'give' or feel tearing as the injury is sustained and there may be bleeding, bruising and swelling. Often however, there is localized cramp caused by muscle spasm in the injured part and the problem gradually resolves with time and treatment. A more insidious problem arises when muscles become chronically tense due, perhaps, to constant repetition of certain movements. Psychological factors such as emotional stress, fear and anxiety can also lead to unconscious tightening and tensing of muscles. Environmental factors, especially exposure to cold can have a similar effect. In these situations, *trigger points* may form. A trigger point is described as a 'knot' of contracted, tense, bunched muscle fibres which, when stimulated ('triggered'), generate a characteristic and familiar pattern of pain. Trigger points can also arise due to damage or dysfunction in adjacent vertebral structures with which the muscle is connected and so the situation may be quite complicated. Pain due to muscle and tendon strain may be treated in a variety of ways, including the application of hot and cold packs, medication, specific exercises, physiotherapy and massage.

Ligament damage can be a cause of serious back pain and it almost always occurs as a result of an accidental event. Instances in which the ligaments of the back may sustain damage include heavy falls and blows and twisting movements such as might occur playing sport or as a result of a road accident. A ligament may be overstretched or, more severely, sustain a partial or total tear. The pain involved can be extremely severe, necessitating calling for emergency medical help. The patient will usually require admittance to hospital to evaluate the nature of the damage. Severe ligament tears may require surgical repair and even if the damage is less serious, healing can be prolonged. The person is likely to need prescription medication in order to deal with the pain and possibly other treatments such as physiotherapy.

7. Vulnerability to Back Pain and Lifestyle Risk Factors

As noted previously, 8 out of 10 people experience back pain at some stage in their life. In addition, surveys reveal that at any one time, half of those questioned will report an occurrence of back pain within the preceding 12 months. It is widely recognized that the greatest risk factor is any previous incidence. Women are at a slightly higher overall risk than men and the reasons for this are not altogether clear. It is possible that pregnancy, childbirth and the general care of small children, which inevitably involves a great deal of bending and lifting, coupled with a greater risk of *osteoporosis* in later life, may account for some of this greater vulnerability.

Pregnancy certainly imposes a risk with many expectant mothers reporting some back pain, especially during the later months. The combination of the increasing weight of the baby and the uterus, coupled with displacement of internal organs and an expanding ribcage, leads to a change in the loading forces exerted on the spine and a shift in the body's usual centre of gravity. Additional hormonal changes, particularly during late pregnancy when the body is becoming prepared for labour, cause a general relaxation of muscles and ligaments. These may easily become fatigued, stretched or strained and hence a focus of pain.

The best way of avoiding or minimizing the likelihood of back pain is to be fit and active before conception and to continue with a healthy lifestyle as pregnancy proceeds. A fit and supple body and especially abdominal muscles that are well toned, all help to support the additional burden of weight at the front and to lessen the effects on the spine. It is also best to keep pregnancy weight gain under control and to avoid prolonged standing, especially in the latter stages. When standing, keeping the feet slightly apart to spread the weight is a helpful strategy. Good, supportive shoes with a broad, low heel are advisable and some women find it helpful to wear a sacral belt to provide additional support. Staying active combined with periods of rest are recommended and there are several exercises designed specifically to help during pregnancy. Walking, swimming, yoga and Pilates are among other beneficial activities that can be undertaken during this period. Due to the extra loading on the spine during pregnancy, it is essential to be particularly careful about bending and twisting movements and to avoid lifting. As pregnancy weight increases, it can be helpful to sleep on one's side, perhaps with the support of a pillow at the back and/or one between the knees as both these measures help to support the spine.

Perhaps surprisingly, *obesity* does not appear, on its own, to increase the risk of first-time incidence of back pain. However, it becomes a significant factor in preventing recurrence and so the best advice is to lose excess weight, if necessary. This has beneficial effects not only for the spine but also for the joints and for overall health and well-being.

Height is significant, with tall people being at greater risk of back pain than those who are of average height or who are short. This is simply down to the mechanics of a greater loading force, particularly on the lower spine. Of course, height is something that lies entirely outside individual control but a tall person may wish to be more than ordinarily 'back aware' and take extra care to prevent problems from arising.

It has long been known that certain specific conditions that cause back pain, such as spondylosis (spinal arthritis) and ankylosing spondylitis, carry genetic links. This means that if one family member is affected, there is higher risk of the condition affecting close relatives. But more recent research has suggested that genes may play a greater part in more generalized forms of back pain than was previously suspected. One of the groups of genes that appear to be involved are those that code for *collagen*, the tough protein substance found in *connective tissue, bone cartilage, tendons* and *skin*. It seems that some people possess genes that make a weaker form of collagen than is present in others and this has implications for their *spinal joints* and more particularly, for the *intervertebral discs*. Once again, there is nothing an individual can do about his or her genetic inheritance but if there is a family incidence of, for example, *degenerative disc disease*, it is wise to adopt a precautionary and protective approach to back care.

As noted above, obesity is a risk factor for recurrent back pain and of course, there is an inevitable relationship between diet (and exercise) and being overweight. People who eat a diet that is high in saturated animal fat and who undertake little exercise are not only more likely to be overweight but also at risk of *atheroma* or *atherosclerosis*. These conditions are characterized by a 'hardening' and narrowing of the arteries due to a build-up of fatty deposits circulating in the bloodstream. Circulation is impaired, and this is further exacerbated by smoking. Not only is there a risk of angina, heart attack and stroke but also there are negative effects upon the spine and more particularly upon the intervertebral discs. There exists a growing body of evidence to suggest that a reduction in circulation has a direct impact upon the progress of disc degeneration during aging. The increased oxygen and nutrient deprivation that results from lowered blood circulation enhances the likelihood of degenerative disc disease occurring. It follows from all of the above that one of the best ways to protect the back is to eat a healthy diet that is low in saturated fat and combine this with taking regular exercise. Giving up smoking is essential.

Some of the more common and obvious triggers of episodes of back pain include the following:

• Incorrect lifting
• Prolonged, standing, bending or crouching
• Poor posture and slouching while sitting
• Twisting, stretching and repetitive movements
• Muscle tension.

Any or all of these may arise during everyday activities, many of them simply because with the passage of time, most of us become lazy and inattentive in the way that we move and use our bodies! Even the simple act of sneezing or coughing can sometimes provoke back pain in certain circumstances. Occupation may place an individual at greater risk, with manual labour and repetitive tasks, eg working on a production line or at a computer, being frequently cited examples. Among school children one of the greatest identified risk factors is the inappropriate carrying of a heavily loaded bag, usually over one shoulder. Other work-related risks may include long-distance driving or the operation of machinery, in both of which vibration can be a contributory factor. In all cases, tiredness, emotional stress and anxiety make matters worse. Very often, a sudden and acute episode of back pain that seems to come 'out of the blue' is, in fact, the end result of a long build-up period in which there has been continual misuse of the back. Further, when considered entirely dispassionately, it is apparent that in some if not in all instances, the remedy lies with ourselves!

8. Prevention

It is impossible to completely prevent back pain; for instance, we cannot help the fact that we age and that, as we do so, some degeneration of our spine is inevitable. However, by making the decision to become 'back aware', by taking some simple precautions and by adopting a healthy lifestyle we can, at least, lessen the risk and, more importantly, reduce the impact that back pain exerts when it happens.

Some preventative measures have been touched upon already while others could be said to fall under the heading of common sense! Being 'back aware' means applying common sense and above all, thinking before you act and heeding any warning signals that your back is giving you. For instance, if you need to lift a heavy weight, always pause and assess the situation. Is the load in fact too great and should you be seeking assistance or finding some other way to move the object? Remember that there is a considerable difference between the weight that you may be physically capable of moving and the one that you can *safely* lift without risk to your back. Secondly, if you are carrying out some activity, eg digging the garden or driving the car on a long journey, and you become aware of nig-gling feelings of discomfort from your back, *always* stop, change your position and take a break. Ignoring symp-toms is likely to lead to pain and one of the best ways to safeguard your back is to regularly change position, per-haps also incorporating some *gentle* stretching to relieve the discomfort. Thirdly, whatever you are doing, adopt a precautionary approach with a healthy respect for your own (and your back's) limitations!

Try to remain *active*. The key points to remember are that physical *inactivity* is bad for all aspects of health in-cluding that of the back and also, the vast majority of people are able to undertake some form of exercise. It is simply a matter of foregoing the excuses and taking the trouble to get started! The meaning of 'taking exercise' can be misinterpreted; in its simplest form, it merely means becoming more active than you are at present. It does not mean that you have to take up some form of ex-treme sport but just that you are prepared to make some usually minor adjustments to your daily routine to incor-porate more activity. It does not have to be expensive. Going for a walk, dancing to music on the radio, taking the stairs instead of the escalator or lift, playing a ball game with children, throwing a stick for the dog, not to mention many voluntary activities – are all free and all count! Even for those already suffering from a bad back, although it may be hard to believe, being active will help to lessen the pain.

Swimming, cycling, yoga and Pilates are all forms of exercise that help to confer strength and flexibility to the spine although it is best to seek guidance before undertaking these if you already have a back problem to make sure that they are suitable for your particular condition. Tai-Chi, however, is a gentle, helpful form of exercise that is suitable for almost everyone, regardless of age and condition.

Specific exercises

There are a number of simple exercises that can be carried out at home which, over a period of time, help to strengthen the back and enhance flexibility.

Knee bends
Stand with your feet apart, each placed slightly beyond the level of your hip. Keeping your back straight, bend at the knees, slowly going down into a squatting position before returning to the upright stance. Repeat 5 times. If necessary, steady yourself by keeping one hand on the back of a chair.

Wall slides
Stand with your feet slightly apart and with your back flat against a wall. Bend your knees and slowly slide into a crouching position using the wall for support. Count to 5 before returning to the upright position. Repeat 5 times.

Curling and uncurling the spine
Stand upright with feet slightly apart and with your head level, looking straight ahead. Slowly bend your head forwards and down, followed by the back of the

neck. Continue your bend with the upper, middle and lower back until you are fully bent over at the waist and your arms are hanging downwards loosely. Keep your knees straight. Concentrate on each part of the spine, feeling the bend as you go down. Now reverse the process, tightening your abdominal muscles so that your pelvis is tucked under your spine. Repeat 5 times.

Arm raises and deep breathing
Stand upright with your arms at your sides. Slowly raise your arms outwards and upwards away from your body while breathing in deeply, feeling the movement of your diaphragm as your lungs inflate. Lower your arms slowly while releasing your breath to reverse the process. Repeat 5 times.

Rotation
Sit astride a chair facing backwards and lock your legs firmly around the seat. Cross your arms and inhale. Rotate slowly one way from the waist as far as you can go, while letting go of your breath. Inhale again as you return to the forward-facing position and then repeat, this time turning to the other side. Repeat 5 times each way.

Leg raises
Lie flat on your back on a carpeted floor with your legs straight. Keep your arms by your sides with the palms of your hands downwards against the floor. Lift one leg slightly off the floor and hold for a count of 5 before lowering. Repeat with the other leg. Lift each leg alternately, 5 times.

Posture

It is an unfortunate fact that many people unconsciously start to adopt bad postural habits during childhood. It may be that modern Western lifestyles, in which so many people spend prolonged periods sitting down, perhaps working on a computer, watching television or driving a car, favours this trend.

Standing in front of a mirror, all too often we are each confronted by the sight of someone with forward-sloping, hunched shoulders and either a rounded, slightly slouched appearance or a 'sway-back' look, with a slack abdomen hanging down at the front instead of in line with the body's centre of gravity! There is a great deal of confusion about what constitutes a 'good pos-ture' but when asked to think about it, most of us are able to recognize when we have adopted a bad one! We may perhaps have been standing (or sitting), shifting our weight onto one side or slouching and on becoming aware of this, we naturally straighten up and square our shoulders. Simply giving this level of attention to our posture is half the battle although it takes more work than this to correct the bad habits of a lifetime! But it is important to try and attain a better posture more of the time in order to prevent back pain and if pain is already present doing this can make a real difference. It does, however, require perseverance because soft tissues adapt to the habitual wrong position that they have been asked to adopt, perhaps for very many years and are therefore likely to 'complain' and hurt at first when a change begins to be imposed!

When standing

Keep your back straight when standing and hold your body upright; relax your shoulders and hold your head level and in the midline, not bent to one side. You should be looking straight ahead. Try to keep your bottom and abdomen tucked in and become aware of your balance, ensuring that your weight is evenly distributed down each leg to your feet. Your legs should be straight and your feet should not be splayed but pointing forwards. Wear well-fitting shoes with a low heel, which feel supportive and comfortable.

When sitting

Keep your back straight and upright when sitting. Your bottom should be at the back of the chair so that the small of your back is supported. You may need to use a small cushion to provide extra support. Try to sit squarely on your seat bones with your hips level. Ideally, keep your feet flat on the floor so that your knees are at the same level. If the chair is the wrong height for you, so that you cannot keep your feet flat, use a book(s) or something similar to correct this.

Whether sitting or standing, imagine that there is an invisible cord running through your body along the line of the centre of gravity and that it becomes fixed when it emerges through the top of your head. Allow the cord to draw you gently upwards in a straight line, so that your neck and every part of your spine follow on naturally. Soften your neck muscles and nod your head slightly, then gently rock your pelvis to align it with your spine. If standing, bend your knees a little to feel your weight on the balls of your feet. Lastly, shrug your shoulders to relax and release them. If you practice this several times each day, just for a few minutes at a time, then after a while your posture should improve.

When driving

Two factors are important in lessening the risk of back pain occurring as a result of driving. The first is to ensure that the back is properly supported and that the height and position of the seat is correctly adjusted to be right for the driver. Your feet should be able to comfortably reach the pedals without any feeling of strain in the legs or backs of the knees. Secondly, it is imperative that on a long journey, regular breaks are taken during which the driver should get out of the car to change position and relieve any muscular tension. The golden rule is to 'change position at regular intervals'.

When using office desks and chairs, and computers

With regard to office chairs, the principle is the same as for sitting. The height of the chair should be adjusted so that your feet can be placed flat on the floor facing forwards and your upper legs should be level or sloping slightly downwards. You should sit so that your back is fully against the backrest and this needs to provide adequate support for the lower back. If necessary, a small cushion can be used to give additional support. When sitting at your desk with your forearms resting on the surface, your elbows should form a right angle. The correct height for the desk is that which allows for this right angle to be made. When working, you should position your chair fairly close to the desk so that you can comfortably maintain a good sitting posture without bending. Armrests should not hinder your ability to adjust the position of the chair. Even when you are sitting and working in the correct position, remember that stresses will still, inevitably, be exerted upon the neck and upper spine due to the fact that you are bending your head and looking downwards. Hence the golden rule of regularly altering your position should be followed.

The top of the monitor screen should be at an arm's length and level with your eyes when you are looking straight ahead. Keep the text line that you are reading or working on at the top of the screen. When using the keyboard, make sure that your shoulders are relaxed and maintain a right angle through your elbows. Keep your wrists straight. Whatever the form of office work in which you are engaged, get up and move about at reasonable intervals and if you are aware of any stiffness or tension, take steps to remedy this by carrying out *gentle* stretches and bends, or massage the affected part. If you are already subject to back pain and suspect that your working environment is contributing to this, you should seek guidance on how this can best be overcome – do not continue as you are but address the problem.

Incorrect lifting and moving of heavy objects

This is one of the most common causes of back injury and pain. But sometimes, the final problem of 'doing the back in' while lifting is the last event in a series of episodes of misuse, in which silently accumulating damage has been incurred. This is all the more reason to consistently ensure that any lifting attempted is always carried out correctly:

- Whenever possible use lifting aids such as a trolley, luggage wheels or a wheelbarrow to help transport the object.
- Before lifting, stand with your feet a little apart and with one foot placed slightly more forward of the other.
- Allow your legs to take the strain by bending your knees but do not go down into a crouching position.
- Bend your trunk forwards a little at the hips.
- Take a good grasp of the object, keeping the heaviest part towards your body, if applicable. Tighten your abdominal muscles.
- Hold the load at waist level. Do not twist your back or lean sideways. Use your feet to turn your body in the direction in which you wish to go.
- Look up and ahead.
- Straighten your legs as you lift and not beforehand.
- If you are moving an object that is too heavy to lift, always push the load rather than pull it.
- When carrying cases or bags, distribute the weight evenly between both hands. Whenever possible, use a well-fitting, comfortable rucksack or backpack to carry loads.

Diet

Eat a healthy, low-fat diet that includes a wide variety of different foods. Vitamins such as vitamin D and calcium are important for the strength of all bones, including those of the spine and supplements may be helpful for some people. It is important to drink plenty of fluids to ensure that intervertebral discs have the best opportunity to remain fully hydrated.

Beds and sleeping

For many years the advice with regard to back care has been to sleep on a firm or hard mattress, often called an *orthopaedic* mattress. However, the thinking behind this has now changed and more recent evidence suggests that a mattress of *medium firmness* is beneficial. The mattress needs to be able to support the whole weight of the body so that no undue stress is placed upon the spine. A recent innovation is the 'memory foam' type of mattress which, it is claimed, can mould to individual body shape and is supportive of the back. This type of mattress may be especially helpful if two people of widely differing size, shape and weight are sharing the same bed.

If pain is present, lying on one side with a pillow between the knees is often helpful and a pillow at the back gives additional support. Alternatively, some people obtain relief by lying on their back with their lower legs resting on pillows.

9. What to Do When Back Pain Strikes

First aid for acute bad backs

As mentioned elsewhere, most episodes of back pain fall into the category of simple back pain and, in the vast majority of cases, this means that the symptoms gradually subside and improve with time. Unless there is a good reason to suspect otherwise, ie in the absence of any severe trauma or previous medical history that might suggest a different cause, it is probably reasonable to assume that yours is a case of simple back pain. However, as has also been stated, this does not mean that the pain you are experiencing is slight or trivial. It may be anything from mild discomfort to agony and, not surprisingly, the severity of the pain greatly influences people's initial reactions and their coping ability. Here are a few key points to bear in mind when dealing with an acute episode of back pain.

Remain active
If you can, continue with your usual routine, even if it is at a modified level. If this proves impossible, move around as much as you can and keep daytime rest periods to

a minimum. There is good, convincing evidence that prolonged rest is unhelpful and slows recovery.

Modify everyday activities

To get up from a prone position, roll over onto your side in the bed and sit up by pushing with your arm on that side. To stand up, push yourself upright from the bed with your arms to lift your bottom and then straighten your knees. In order to get dressed, do not sit or bend from the waist. Stand with your back flat against a wall for support and put on socks, trousers etc by first raising one leg, then the other, bending at the knee. Avoid sitting down for long periods by getting up as described above but when you do sit, make sure that the chair you use gives very good support. At all times, keep your back straight; do not bend, twist, lift or carry.

Take painkillers

Ordinary, over-the-counter preparations such as *paracetamol* and *ibuprofen* will take the edge off the pain and enable you to move more comfortably.

Apply hot and/or cold packs

Experiment to see which of these brings the most relief. A wheat bag that can be heated in the microwave is ideal but a hot water bottle can be used, provided it is covered. A hot bath is often also soothing and aromatherapy products added to the water may aid relaxation. A pack of frozen peas wrapped in a tea towel makes a handy ice pack and can be used over and over again for that purpose.

Use pillows

In bed, use pillows to obtain a more comfortable sleeping position (as described on page 69). Avoid sleeping during the day.

Practice relaxation

Find a quiet room and either sit or lie down. Close your eyes and breathe out in and out slowly and evenly. Allow your lungs to empty fully with each out-breath by relaxing your chest and diaphragm and pausing for a moment before breathing in again. Focus on your body and check for areas of tension; try to relax them.

Beginning with your feet, concentrate on releasing and letting go of any muscular tension. Your feet should feel heavy and warm when you have finished. Carry on with the process, working up through your lower legs, knees, upper legs, pelvis, trunk, neck, face and head, allowing all the muscles to slacken and relax. You should feel warm and comfortable and your breathing should be even and relaxed the whole time. This exercise in relaxation should help to lessen the discomfort and pain that you are experiencing, even if the pain does not go completely.

Now let go of any intrusive thoughts and cares by deliberately excluding them from your mind. Imagine that you are watching a meadow full of brightly coloured flowers in the sunshine, or a pool with ripples shining in the moonlight or a crystal clear stream gently flowing over pebbles. Alternatively, think of an image that is appropriate for you, perhaps involving some precious memory. With your eyes closed, you may be able to 'see' colours or patterns; watch and enjoy them. Remain like this for 15 to 30 minutes.

If the pain is still intrusive, try a different tack and attempt to regard it in a detached, unemotional way – a process known as *visualization*. Imagine that the pain has a shape, weight and colour, picking those that seem most appropriate to you. As you continue to breathe evenly, imagine that the colour lightens in time to your rhythmic breathing and becomes a pastel shade. Next think about the shape and try to alter it to something more soft and yielding. Likewise with the weight – see if you can make it appear lighter and thinner and more manoeuvrable. Think of it as a soap bubble that can be wafted out of your body. The pain bubble may re-enter but with practice, you will be able to control its activity for more of the time.

Very severe pain
If the pain is very severe and does not improve despite self-help measures or if you are unable to sleep or obtain any relief, it is sensible to obtain expert medical advice.

When to call for help

As stated above, you should in all cases, seek help if you are worried about back pain. But in addition, there are situations in which seeking medical aid is essential:

- The back pain has arisen following a significant and recent blow, accident or trauma – even if it is one which did not seem too important at the time.

- There is swelling and/or inflammation.
- There is an accompanying fever of 38°C/100.4°F.
- The level of pain is increasing substantially.
- The pain is additionally travelling down the leg(s) beyond the knees.
- Pain is additionally present in the chest.
- There is numbness and weakness in the legs.
- There is inability to pass urine or urinary incontinence and/or bowel incontinence.
- There is a previous history of cancer.
- There is lowered immunity due to chemotherapy or other treatment or medical condition.
- The back pain was slight at first but has gradually become more severe, perhaps over several weeks or a longer time period.
- The patient is aged under 20 or over 55 years.
- The patient has been taking prescribed steroid drugs.
- The patient has been using illegal drugs.

10. More Common Medical Conditions that Cause Back Pain

As has already been noted, back pain is usually quite complex and often results from more than one cause or problem. Hence the conditions that cause back pain tend not to fit neatly into categories possessing readily defined limits that can be easily described and classified! Added to this is the fact that there is quite a degree of overlap in the medical terminology that is used in relation to back pain and this can add to the difficulty!

As stated previously, instances of back pain are usually assigned to one of three categories with simple back pain, which is self-limiting and generally has no clearly discernible cause, being responsible for 94% of all cases. In about 5% of cases there is nerve pain due to compression and irritation and the remaining 1% are attributed to some other underlying pathological condition.

The conditions described below certainly account for some of the cases in the 5% and 1% categories but not exclusively. Since many are degenerative and produce, to some degree, quite a wide variation in severity of symptoms depending upon the stage they are at, they may also be responsible for some simple back pain as well. Finally, although they may account for only 6% of back pain, the conditions are not necessarily uncommon or rare in terms of the number of people affected. Due to the overall prevalence of back pain, the actual number of individuals affected may be quite high.

Osteoporosis

Osteoporosis is characterized by a progressive loss of bone tissue, and this is due to the fact that the rate at which material is being reabsorbed greatly outstrips that at which new material can be made and replenished. Osteoporosis affects all bones, not only those of the back, and it leads to a general loss of bone density posing a higher risk of fracture. It is important in relation to back pain because it is a feature of several degenerative disorders of the spine. Some gradual reduction in bone density is a normal factor of aging and one that affects older people of both sexes. This is a contributor, along with thinning and hardening of the intervertebral discs, to the slow reduction in height that takes place as we age. However, osteoporosis is a more extreme condition in which there is considerable thinning of bones and greatly increased fragility. It can be a silent condition; one which may only come to light when a minor, insignificant fall results in a bone fracture, often of the hip.

There may be few other signs and symptoms but if these do arise, they include a rapid loss of height and increased spinal curvature (*kyphosis*) as well as backache. In women, there is a direct link with the sudden decline in the level of the hormone oestrogen, experienced after the menopause. Hence post-menopausal women are the group most at risk, particularly those who are of slight build. Other risk factors include anorexia during adolescence and young adulthood (the period when life-long bone density is being achieved), smoking, poor nutrition and especially a low calcium intake, malabsorption conditions and chronic digestive disorders. Also, certain hereditary factors, Paget's disease of bone, osteomalacia, Cushing's syndrome, prolonged corticosteroid treatment and slight build and fair hair. Women who have undergone radiotherapy treatment for ovarian cancer are also at greater risk. Once diagnosed, treatment involves ensuring that a good diet – containing plenty of calcium, vitamin D and minerals – is eaten, with supplements prescribed if necessary. Also, bone-strengthening and mineralization preparations may be prescribed, eg biphosphonates. Treatment of any back pain associated with the condition is likely to include analgesic medication, physiotherapy and tailor-made, gentle exercises undertaken with specialist supervision.

Spondylosis

Spondylosis is a term as much as it is a condition and it means degenerative changes or 'wear and tear' affecting the spine (from *spondylos* the Greek word for 'vertebra'). It refers to the *normal* degeneration that takes place with aging and the most significant aspect of it is that in any particular individual, it may or may not be responsible for back pain! Spondylosis includes the bony projections known as *osteophytes* that may grow in and around spinal joints and intervertebral discs due to remodelling, as well as degenerative changes affecting the discs themselves. It ably illustrates why x-rays are now used cautiously rather than routinely in modern investigative medicine, when trying to establish the cause of back pain. In the past, the existence of spondylosis on an x-ray of the spine would frequently have been seen as the cause of an individual's back pain. But medical thinking has now changed and the reason for this is that extensive research has revealed that spondylosis is commonly present in people who are pain-free. Indeed, there can be discernible spondylosis-type changes apparent on the x-rays of people as young as 18 years old while half of those aged 50 will have the condition. But significantly, many of these people are, and remain, free from back pain.

However, the converse is not necessarily true and it cannot be said that spondylosis is not responsible for the back pain of any particular individual. What all this does highlight is the limited usefulness of ascertaining cause when what is important is the manner in which back pain is treated and managed. No treatment is needed for spondylosis that is not causing problems. Treatment for pain is likely to include a combination of analgesic and, possibly, anti-inflammatory drugs and muscle-relaxants as well as physiotherapy and the wearing of a neck or lumbar support brace, depending upon the location of the pain. Surgery is rarely required and possibly only indicated if there is pressure on a nerve that is causing severe symptoms, such as muscle weakness or problems with the control of the bladder or bowel.

Degenerative spondylolisthesis/ collapsed vertebrae

Spondylolisthesis describes a condition in which a lumbar vertebra (usually L4 or L5) has slipped forwards (or rarely backwards) so as to be out of alignment with the rest of the spine. The condition develops slowly as a result of the gradual elongation of the bony neural arch between the two articular processes of the affected vertebrae. This eventually results in the instability, and then failure, of the bony 'catches' provided by the facet joints that lock the spinal segments together. This failure enables increased, abnormal movement of the overlying vertebra resulting in slippage. There may be accompanying formation of *osteophytes* and spinal stenosis, with a risk of nerve root compression and sciatica and, in extreme cases, impairment of bladder or bowel function. Symptoms include low back pain of varying degrees of severity, stiffness, numbness, tingling and weakness. The condition is more common in women and usually affects people aged over 50 years. It arises as a combination of spondylosis and spinal osteoarthritis, accompanied by disc degeneration. Osteoporosis may be a contributory factor.

First-line treatment involves the use of analgesic and anti-inflammatory drugs and, possibly, physiotherapy and the wearing of a back brace to support the spine. A specific exercise regime aimed at building up muscle strength, particularly in the abdominal region to support the back, may be recommended. In more severe cases where there is nerve root involvement, spinal injections

79

may be considered. Surgery to effect nerve decompression and/or vertebral fusion may be needed in particular instances, especially if other treatments have failed to provide relief or if there is impaired function of the bladder or bowel. In many people, the condition may progress of its own accord to a more stable position in older age, due to the normal hardening that occurs within intervertebral discs. As the discs dry out and turn fibrous, there may be an effective fusion between the two vertebrae that are responsible, fixing the slippage and so lessening the problems caused.

Conditions affecting intervertebral discs

Disc degeneration and dehydration

Disc degeneration and dehydration is a natural and universal consequence of aging. As a result of a gradual loss of fluid due to a decline in the efficiency of *intradiscal fluid exchange* combined with other changes, discs eventually become almost entirely fibrous in nature. They become thinner and there is a loss of the flexibility that was present in youth. In many people, the condition is not painful and the most that they may experience is loss of flexibility and a degree of stiffness.

In the course of this progressive pattern of degeneration, one or more discs may *bulge* under the pressure exerted upon the spine during movement. This may cause pain and can be a precursor to a *prolapse* of the disc. The origins of the pain are twofold. The outer wall of the disc (*annular fibrosus*) is supplied with nerves from the

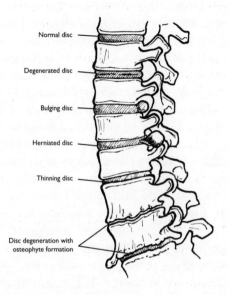

Fig 9 Some examples of disc problems

segmental nerves and *dorsal root ganglion* at each level. Mechanical distension caused by the bulging may cause nerve fibres to fire and generate pain signals. In addition, the bulging may sometimes compress a nearby nerve root in which case, *referred pain* may be experienced in the areas to which the nerve extends. A significant bulge is more likely to cause pain than a minor one but this also depends, to some extent, upon the location of the problem within the vertebral column. Problems with discs, whether bulges or *herniation,* are far more likely to affect middle-aged people between the ages of 30 and 50 years.

81

This is the 'in between' period, during which intervertebral discs are gradually losing the full plumpness of youth but have not yet become totally dry and fibrous.

Since disc dehydration is a natural process, it does not require treatment unless a disc is bulging and causing pain. The best ways to prevent problems developing and to maximize disc heath are twofold. Firstly, if applicable, give up smoking. Tobacco smoke reduces the amount of oxygen and nutrients reaching the discs in the blood circulation and this favours the process of dehydration and degeneration. Secondly, remain active and maintain a strong back by regularly taking exercise.

Treatment for more severe discogenic pain caused by bulging is likely to involve analgesic and anti-inflammatory preparations in the first instance. Physiotherapy and specific exercises may also help and/or chiropractic and acupuncture. If there is nerve root involvement, other medication may be prescribed. Surgery is rarely a solution and then only as a last resort when other options have failed.

Prolapsed, herniated, protruded, ruptured or slipped disc

As may be seen from the heading, a number of words are commonly used, practically interchangeably, to describe what is essentially one condition! So before beginning to discuss what it means to have a prolapsed disc, it is first useful to say a little about this terminology. Firstly, although 'slipped disc' is a popular, descriptive phrase and one that is familiar to many people, it not only lacks any medical credentials but is also entirely misleading since, contrary to widely held belief, discs do not and indeed cannot 'slip'! Nevertheless, an idea persists that a slipped disc means one that has physically moved either forwards, backwards or sideways from its true position in the spine. But this is never the case and is a physical impossibility. The other four terms are medical ones but, to add to the confusion, each may be used in differing ways by different doctors! 'Ruptured' and 'herniated' are usually reserved for complete disc breakdown (as described below) but 'prolapsed' and 'protruded' may either be used in relation to this extreme or with reference to degrees of bulging, as outlined above. Hence it can be seen that prolapse in relation to intervertebral discs incorporates a scale of possible problems. These range from slight bulging with or without pain to partial or complete rupture involving severe pain and other possible symptoms.

As has been seen, discs degenerate and become weaker with increasing age. This process not only affects the gel-like *nucleus pulposus* in the centre of each disc but also the outer, ligamentous 'tyre', the *annulus fibrosus* (*see* Fig 5 on page 39). It is this weakening and increased flaccidness of the outer ring that enables the nucleus pulposus to bulge outwards against and into the outer wall, when subjected to compression. Sometimes the wall gradually cracks beneath the pressure and one or more fissures, known as *annular tears* arise into which the nuclear material is forced. While the outermost layers hold, the prolapse is contained and although it may cause pain, it is incomplete. But a more extreme situation, one of complete herniation, arises when the tearing penetrates right

83

through the disc wall enabling nuclear material to be extruded under pressure. All too often, this causes accompanying compression and irritation of one or more segmental nerves or the nuclear material may even find its way through the fibrous layer of the *posterior longitudinal ligament* to penetrate the *spinal canal*, allowing possible interference with the *spinal cord*. Apart from the mechanical pressure exerted, the nuclear material is also highly irritating, the more so because it too has undergone degenerative change. Enzymes cause denaturation of the proteins within the nucleus making the material highly inflammatory and irritating to the *dural sheath* and other delicate membranes lining the nerves, This combination of leakage and irritation tends to cause swelling, further exacerbating the pressure and duress to which the nerves are subjected.

Whatever the extent of the herniation, pain is commonly present and it may be both local and referred. Localized pain depends upon the position of the affected disc within the spinal column but referred pain depends upon the distribution of the nerve that is subject to irritation. Some 95% of herniations arise in lumbar discs with the cervical spine (the neck) accounting for most of the remainder. It is rare for thoracic vertebrae to be involved as the range of movement (and hence compression of the discs) is more limited in this region of the spine. Pain is often described as sharp or cutting. In the lumbar spine, it arises in the lower back and often extends into the buttocks, thighs and possibly down into the foot, usually on one side (*see* 'Sciatica' on page 87).

There may even be numbness and a degree of paralysis in the foot, known as 'foot-drop'. In the cervical spine, pain affects the neck and may radiate into the shoulders and arms, again often on one side. In the rare case of prolapse of a thoracic disc, pain is experienced in the mid-back and possibly in the chest. Nerve root pressure and/or pressure on the spinal cord may cause muscle spasms and degrees of muscular paralysis and, rarely, interference with the control the bladder, bowel or sexual organs (*cauda equina syndrome*). (It should be noted that *sacral nerves* are susceptible to pressure from herniated lumbar discs because, although they leave the spinal cord through exit holes in the fused sacrum, they then run through the lumbar spine within the cauda equina.) Pain may restrict the range of normal movement in the back and if the legs are affected, the ability to walk can also be impaired.

The symptoms of herniation may arise gradually or suddenly. If gradual, the pain is sometimes reported as beginning in the morning and then worsening if it travels down the leg. In other cases the pain arises suddenly, often following an awkward lift, bend or twisting movement. The person may even feel a tearing sensation, believed to be damage occurring to ligaments and/or muscles. In these instances, this final episode usually follows years in which silent degeneration and weakening has been taking place, unsuspected by the person concerned. The pain may be so acute that for a time, the person cannot bend the back in any direction or even fully straighten up. He or she may be bent to one side and weight-bearing may be almost unbearable. Coughing and sneezing can exacerbate the pain. Disc prolapse may also arise as a result of an accidental injury to the back such as a fall, blow or road traffic accident.

Although these symptoms are undoubtedly alarming as well as painful, provided that there is no sign of severe nerve root pressure, spinal cord compression or cauda equina syndrome, there is no need to seek emergency medical help. But it is advisable to call the doctor for advice and probably to make an appointment. Diagnosis is usually made by means of a physical examination and discussion of the sequence of events and previous medical history. It is often possible to determine the position of a suspect disc by these means, although a doctor may wish to obtain scan or x-ray results for confirmation.

It is normal procedure for a conservative approach to treatment to be adopted. This may include a minimal period of bed-rest although, as with most back problems, it is now considered better for light, gentle activity to be resumed as soon as possible. Analgesic and anti-inflammatory medication is usually required and in due course, physiotherapy, specific exercises, acupuncture, chiropractic and osteopathy are further avenues that may be considered helpful. Surgery would only be considered as a last resort and it is worth remembering that most disc herniations improve and tend to resolve themselves, within a period of 6 to 12 months.

In the event of severe nerve root pain and possible weakness or paralysis in certain muscles, lack of sensation and loss of tendon reflexes, strong analgesic and anti-inflammatory medication will certainly be prescribed and there may be a need for onward referral for such as some form of spinal injection. Symptoms of spinal cord and/or cauda equina involvement include muscular spasms, loss of sensation or disturbance in the area of the groin and rectum and/or thighs, loss or reduction in control of bladder or bowel function and numbness or degrees of paralysis in the limbs (usually the legs). These are known as 'red flag' symptoms (*see* page 131) and, if present, immediate medical treatment is required (usually surgery) to relieve the pressure on the nerves (*see* 'Cauda equina syndrome' on page 88).

Sciatica

Sciatica describes a particular form of pain caused by activation of the sciatic nerve, arising as a result of pinching and pressure causing irritation and inflammation. Although generally thought of as a condition in its own right, sciatica is more correctly a syndrome caused by a problem elsewhere, usually in the lumbar spine. Hence although its characteristic feature is leg pain, this generally accompanies low back pain rather than occurring in isolation. The sciatic nerve is the major nerve running down each leg. It descends from the base of the spine along the back of the thigh and it incorporates a number of nerve roots issuing from the lower part of the spinal cord. Sciatica usually occurs on one side and pain is felt in the lower back, the buttock and down into the leg, sometimes reaching the foot. The pain may be felt on the outer part of the leg or foot and there may be stiffness, weakness, numbness or a sensation of 'pins-and-needles' in the affected areas. The precise distribution of pain depends on which nerve roots are affected. (An essentially similar set of symptoms affecting the neck, shoulder and arm on one side may arise if the source of the problem is higher up in the spine but it is less common and does not have a specific name.) The pain can be severe and stabbing and movement of the leg tends to exacerbate the problem by further stretching the nerve. Weight-bearing may be difficult or almost impossible and may only be achieved by holding the leg bent. This can lead to unequal contraction of muscles, forcing the hips out of alignment.

A common cause of sciatica is a bulging or herniated disc but inflammation of facet joints may also be involved. Rare causes include ankylosing spondylitis or a spinal tumour. Treatment may include a minimal period of bed-rest until the acute symptoms subside but essentially it is now considered best to try and maintain or resume activity as soon as possible. Analgesic and anti-inflammatory medication is usually prescribed to help control the pain. Physiotherapy, osteopathy, chiropractic and acupuncture may prove helpful in the longer term. Spinal injections (epidural or nerve root blocking) may be needed if pain is extremely severe and disabling. Surgery (discetomy or microdiscetomy) may be considered eventually as a last resort to relieve the pressure on the nerve. But the most usual approach, especially to begin with, is to try and manage the pain by non-invasive means.

Cauda equina syndrome
Cauda equina syndrome is a rare condition but it is included here because, as with sciatica, when it does occur it is usually in connection with a herniated lumbar disc.

However, other possible causes include spinal injury, a viral infection in the spine and certain congenital conditions such as spina bifida. As noted above, this condition involves the fantail of nerves at the base of the spinal cord and it may cause a wide variety of symptoms. These include a loss of sensation, numbness, tingling, 'pins-and-needles' and degrees of muscular paralysis affecting the buttocks, groin, legs and feet. There may also be a loss or reduction in control of the bladder and bowel and impotence. A person who notices any of these 'red flag' symptoms (*see* page 131) should always seek medical advice. In some cases the condition is a temporary one caused by damage to the myelin sheath surrounding the affected nerves. This will usually resolve although recovery may take some time and should always be medically monitored. More severe cases, in which the nerves have become damaged, will nearly always require corrective surgery and there is a far greater chance of making a good recovery with early diagnosis and treatment. If left untreated, cauda equina syndrome can result in permanent disability and paralysis.

Spinal stenosis

Spinal stenosis refers to the abnormal narrowing of one or more of the spaces occupied by the spinal cord and its associated nerves, usually in one particular area. The narrowing may affect the central spinal canal which houses the spinal cord or one or more of the intervertebral foramina (lateral canal stenosis) through which run the segmental spinal nerves.

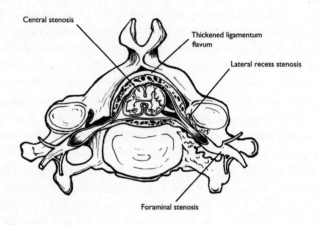

Central stenosis

Thickened ligamentum flavum

Lateral recess stenosis

Foraminal stenosis

Fig 10 Spinal stenosis

Spinal stenosis commonly occurs as a result of the degenerative changes accompanying aging. It may be caused by changes in discs, with encroachment into the canal spaces or by the growth of osteophytes from facet joints or other parts of the vertebrae or, quite frequently, by a combination of all of these. Sometimes, the large, yellow ligamentum flavum becomes thickened and scarred as a result of degeneration in discs and vertebrae and this causes further narrowing. In some cases, the spinal canal may be congenitally narrow at birth and while this may not be a problem in youth, it makes affected individuals vulnerable to spinal stenosis in later life.

Spinal stenosis usually affects the lumbar region and generally progresses slowly. Typically the symptoms are worse with standing and walking and relieved by sitting down. This is because the position of the lumbar spine when seated naturally tends to open up the spinal canal. Common symptoms include lower back and leg pain or sensations of tingling, heaviness or numbness affecting the lower limbs. People affected may discover that they are only able to walk a progressively shorter distance before pain, unsteadiness and loss of balance forces them to stop and sit down. Those affected typically adopt a stooped posture and the condition can be quite severely disabling. The symptoms are caused by *neurogenic claudication* in which the circulation of blood to lumbar nerves is reduced due to the narrowing of the spinal canal. Lateral canal stenosis may occasionally arise on its own with no spinal canal involvement and in this case, pain may be restricted to the distribution of a single nerve root running down into the leg. But the general pattern of symptoms is the same as described above, being worse with upright activity and relieved by sitting down.

Treatment in the first instance usually comprises analgesic and anti-inflammatory medication to deal with pain. Physiotherapy, specific exercises, changes in posture and sleeping position, chiropractic and wearing a back brace may all prove helpful. Steroid injections into the canal space to reduce inflammation may sometimes be considered as a short-term measure to provide relief. Targeted, combined anaesthetic and corticosteroid injections into the epidural space or nerve root blocking may be considered suitable for some patients, but spinal decompression surgery may be the final option to provide longer-term relief. However, this would only be considered after other methods have been tried and it involves a thorough physical examination and detailed imaging (MRI scanning) before surgery can be carried out. The structures that are commonly removed in this type of surgery are osteophytes, small sections of lamina (bony arch) from offending vertebrae, and bulging or herniated discs. Once obstructions are removed, normal blood flow is re-established and the restored canal space is wide enough to again accommodate the nerve without the risk of compression.

Sacroiliac joint disorder/dysfunction

The sacroiliac joint can be a source of pain due to strain of the strong ligaments in this area. Symptoms include pain and stiffness and this may be severe, affecting the inner and upper part of the buttock on the involved side. Pain may also be referred into the groin and down the leg and there may be muscle spasm and difficulty in walking. Symptoms also may arise on both sides in some cases. In people severely affected, there may be a slight rotation of the pelvis on the affected side causing an apparent minimal difference in leg length and this contributes to the difficulty experienced in walking. It can be difficult to diagnose this condition and this is usually achieved by means of physical examinations and a detailed study of the patient's medical history. In some cases, pain-blocking injections into the affected region may be carried out, both as a treatment and as a confirmation of the likely source of the problem. Due to the severity of the pain, prescribed analgesic medication will almost certainly be required with physiotherapy and manipulation being other helpful means of dealing with an acute attack. If symptoms are frequently recurrent, fibroproliferative therapy or prolotherapy may be helpful (*see* page 161). Rarely, the sacroiliac joint can be a focus of inflammation (sacroilitis), which is connected with some underlying disorder such as Crohn's disease, ulcerative colitis, psoriasis, seronegative spondylo-arthropathy or ankylosing spondylitis. In the latter case and especially if the patient is a young person, sacroilitis may be the first sign of this disorder. Symptoms of sacroilitis include low back pain and stiffness, especially on rising in the morning. Blood tests and possibly an MRI scan may form part of the investigations that are likely to be carried out. Treatment will depend upon underlying cause but is likely to include anti-inflammatory and analgesic medication and possibly antibiotics in the first instance.

Ankylosing spondylitis (AS)

Ankylosing spondylitis is a progressive, inflammatory, rheumatic disease affecting the spine, sacroliac joints and hips. It is far more common in males and although it can arise at any time, typical age of onset is between 10 and 40 years. It rarely arises suddenly and symptoms usually begin gradually and worsen with time. In the early stages, there is lower back pain and stiffness, especially upon arising in the morning or following a period of rest. Later the disease progresses to involve the whole spine and the inflammation may cause vertebrae to fuse together so that the structure becomes rigid or forward bending. Areas of fusion are often quite brittle and susceptible to injury, particularly fracture. AS is diagnosed by means of physical examinations, blood tests and studying the detailed medical history of the patient. This often reveals that the person is suffering from a form of arthritis affecting other joints in the body. AS is a painful, debilitating condition and one that confers a risk of depression and at an advanced stage, may affect kidney function. Hence regular testing of urine samples may be required to monitor kidney function.

Although there is no cure, treatment and self-help measures can enable a sufferer to manage and alleviate the worst of the symptoms. Many patients find heat, in the form of hot baths and heat pads to be helpful in alleviating pain and stiffness. Non-steroidal anti-inflammatory medication is generally prescribed and, sometimes, drugs that lower the body's immune response are used as an alternative. These are also helpful in lessening inflammation. Steroid injections may be used, generally as a short-term treatment and with caution. Physiotherapy and massage are other mainstays of treatment, along with specific back-strengthening exercises, but these must always be carried out under the supervision of a fully trained specialist. Sufferers are usually recommended to remain active, with walking and swimming being particularly useful forms of exercise for those with this condition. Activities that jar or stress the spine, such as running, should be avoided.

The cause is unknown but there is good evidence for a genetic link with the condition tending to run in families. Hence individuals with one or more affected relatives are particularly advised to adopt a healthy, active lifestyle to lessen the initial impact, should symptoms arise. It is very important to avoid smoking. Spinal supports in the form of a back brace or belt may help a sufferer to remain active. Due to the progressive nature of AS, psychological support for sufferers is important, whether this takes the form of specialist help or encouragement and understanding from friends and family. Emphasis should be placed on what can still be achieved and in setting realistic goals for the future so that the person can continue to have the best possible quality of life within the limits imposed by the condition.

Ligament hypermobility

Ligament hypermobility is a syndrome that most commonly affects women following pregnancy and childbirth. It is natural for ligaments in the pelvic region to relax as pregnancy progresses in preparation for childbirth but in some women, they may fail to tighten up again after the baby has been born. These ligaments, especially those associated with the sacroiliac joint, then fail to hold pelvic structures correctly in place, allowing a greater than normal degree of movement. Symptoms of hypermobility include pain and this may affect one or both hips and the lower back. It may be severe and interfere with the ability to move and walk. Treatment includes analgesic drugs to alleviate pain coupled with physiotherapy and specific exercises designed to strengthen the structures in the affected area. Some patients may benefit from fibroproliferative or prolotherapy (*see* page 161).

Coccydinia

Coccydinia is a fairly common form of low back pain and describes pain originating in the *coccyx* or tailbone. Women are at greater risk although men may also be affected. In women, the most common cause is bruising and trauma to the coccyx during childbirth. Others include a sudden, accidental injury as a result of a fall or blow, which may also cause a fracture or dislocation. However, similar damage can also be caused through certain, repetitive sporting activities, such as cycling and horse riding, in which the coccyx is subject to sustained pressure. The degree of intensity and nature of the pain experienced depends, to some extent, upon the cause. It varies from a dullish ache to an acute, sharp pain in the event of a fracture. In all cases and perhaps not surprisingly, the pain is made worse by sitting and the person may find it difficult to obtain a comfortable position.

Before treatment can be started it is necessary to discover the nature of the damage and this may require x-rays to ascertain whether there has been a break or dislocation. Admittance to hospital for corrective surgery may be needed and in all cases analgesic medication is likely to be prescribed for pain relief. Injections of combined local anaesthetic and steroid preparations may help some patients and these usually require attendance at an outpatient clinic. Physiotherapy and osteopathy may also prove helpful. A supportive, well-padded cushion is a necessity for someone suffering from coccydinia and sitting on hard chairs should be avoided until recovery is complete.

Common, structural anomalies that may be connected with back pain

A surprisingly high number of people show structural anomalies in their spine and many of these are believed to be congenital and/or to arise during growth. In the majority of cases they appear to cause no harm and are usually discovered coincidentally. Hence their involvement in the generation of back pain, whether in general terms or on an individual basis, may be hard to ascertain. In most cases, an identified anomaly of this nature in an adult does not need treatment or monitoring and any form of intervention or correction is rare. However, if a structural anomaly is identified in a child, precautionary monitoring as growth proceeds is likely to be recommended so that any progression of the anomaly can be picked up at an early stage. When it is required, intervention usually takes the form of corrective, specially formulated postural exercises. Surgery (spinal bracing) is rarely needed and then only in the event of a definitive disorder being present.

Transitional vertebrae
Sometimes it appears that a vertebra lying at a junction between different regions of the spine has suffered a

form of 'identity crisis' during development and has adopted a somewhat different shape and form. The usual site where this occurs is at the sacral/lumbar junction. The 5th lumbar may fuse with the sacral segments below or, alternatively, the 1st sacral may be detached to form an extra lumbar vertebra. These so-called transitional vertebrae arise during foetal development. There are no known problems associated with this spinal arrangement and it is normal for the individuals in whom it occurs.

Spina bifida occulta

Spina bifida occulta describes a relatively common developmental anomaly affecting L5, in which the bony neural arch does not fuse in the centre. It is entirely harmless and is usually identified during routine screening in pregnancy. On no account should it be confused with the far more serious condition of spina bifida.

Lordosis

Lordosis is the term given to the natural hollowing or concavity that occurs in the cervical and lumbar spine. The term *lumbar lordosis* may be used to describe a greater than usual hollowing of the lower back in which the forward curvature of the spine is exaggerated.

Kyphosis

Kyphosis is the name given to the natural convexity of the profile of the thoracic spine. It may also be used to describe a more pronounced rounded or humpback appearance in which the backward curvature of the thoracic spine is excessive. Kyphosis in old age may produce a stooped appearance and it is often brought about by loss of height due to osteoporosis, perhaps compounded by compression fracture. This requires special treatment, probably combining analgesic pain relief and dietary changes and supplementation with bone-strengthening preparations such as biphosphonates. Kyphosis is not normally associated with back pain but if it first arises in adult life or in middle age, monitoring and further investigation may be needed, particularly if it is progressive. Kyphosis in children must always be monitored and investigated and it can be an early sign of Scheuermann's disease (*see* page 108).

Scoliosis or curvature of the spine

Scoliosis is the name given to a lateral or sideways bend in the spine. It usually affects the thoracic spine or the junction between this and the lumbar spine. In rare cases it may be confined to the lumbar spine alone. A slight variation is relatively common and it is not normally a cause of back pain. One type of lateral deviation, producing a wide, gentle curve throughout the whole length of the spine, is most commonly associated with a tilted pelvis (*see* next page), which is itself caused by a slight difference in leg length. In adults a slight scoliosis does not usually require treatment unless associated pain is present, attributable to the condition. However, as aging progresses the curvature may become more pronounced and in this case, treatment in the form of postural exercises would be the most likely recommendation, possibly combined with wearing a back support or brace. Surgical spinal bracing or any other corrective surgery is rarely performed. However, in a child showing developmental and structural scoliosis, monitoring and treatment is far more likely to be required. In a child, the scoliosis is much more obvious when he or she bends forward when there will be an evident rib hump. A specialist is likely to recommend corrective postural exercises in the first instance. Surgery is viewed very much as a last resort and is only carried out if the degree of curvature has progressed to an angle greater than 45 degrees.

Tilted pelvis/pelvic obliquity

Tilted pelvis is a relatively common condition that usually arises gradually and is generally associated with a slight difference in the length of each leg. This disparity, known as an *anatomical leg length discrepancy* may only be minute, amounting to less than a few millimetres and the person may be unaware of its existence. Even so, the effect can be considerable since the person unconsciously compensates by putting more weight on one side, to correct the imbalance on the loading of the spine. It is this that ultimately causes pelvic obliquity and this may then generate low back pain and tenderness in the *iliopsoas muscles*. (These muscles, comprising the *iliacus* and *psoas*, are the strong muscles that flex the hip and allow the leg to be extended in front of the body. They are deep-seated muscles lying in front of the hip and attaching to the thigh bone by means of the *iliopsoas tendon*.) If left untreated, the problem can progress to interfere with mobility and cause quite severe pain with walking. In some affected persons, but by no means in all, there is the visible appearance of being lopsided. In order to diagnose the condition, a physical examination is carried out and measurements of leg length are obtained, while the patient is supine and also while seated.

Treatment methods include analgesic medication and spinal manipulation that must be performed by a chiropractor or other trained specialist. Heat, by means of hot packs applied externally to relieve muscle spasm is often soothing. A further option is myofascial release treatment (MFR). This is a specialized form of massage that should only be performed by a trained practitioner and it is aimed directly at affected muscles. Tilted pelvis may arise in relation to lifestyle with prolonged sitting, or walking or running for long distances potentially posing a higher risk. Chronic hydration, in which tissues are overfilled with fluid is a further risk factor and if present, requires further investigation and treatment.

Spinal injuries

Whiplash
Whiplash is the name given to a particular type of injury involving the head, neck and upper spine. It is most commonly caused by a motor vehicle accident in which the vehicle comes to a sudden stop due to impact. In this situation the head, which is a heavy structure balanced upon a highly mobile neck, is first thrown violently backwards and then forwards under considerable forces of acceleration and deceleration. Various structures may be torn and damaged including discs, facet joints, ligaments and muscles. In half of all cases, the source of whiplash

pain lies within the ligamentous capsules of the facet joints and their articular surfaces. Symptoms include a very stiff neck with pain that may be both acute and severe, especially with movement. A stabbing pain in the head, sometimes radiating into the shoulder, headache and dizziness may also be present. Symptoms may not always arise immediately but can develop some 2 to 3 days after the accident. Typically, a person is guarded in his or her movements and holds the head on one side. Treatment involves analgesic and anti-inflammatory medication in the first instance and application of heat pads may also be soothing. Once the acute symptoms have subsided, physiotherapy is likely to be needed. Unfortunately, due to damage sustained in the facet joints, there is a risk of eventual development of cervical spondylosis with symptoms of stiffness and pain and sometimes a sensation of grinding or clicking. The joints and muscles may feel tense and hard, relieved by rubbing the neck. Other symptoms that may arise include lack of concentration, tiredness, headaches, a feeling of heaviness in the head, pain in the teeth, ringing in the ears and vision disturbance. Emotional stress, tension and anxiety are likely to exacerbate the symptoms. Treatment methods are similar to those employed in an acute attack with physiotherapy and possibly wearing a neck support, forming an important part of managing the condition.

Spinal fractures

Spinal fractures are usually caused by trauma and most commonly as a result of a fall or blow to the back, sustained during a road traffic accident or while engaged in certain active sports. Those most at risk are people who engage in sports such as rugby, football, gymnastics, skiing, horse-riding or any other activity where there is a possibility of a fall from a height. Some occupations may also pose a greater risk, particularly those involving hard physical labour as in construction, farming, offshore oil exploration, mining etc. A further 'at risk' group are elderly people with osteoporosis in whom a simple slip or fall may cause a fracture. There are three main types of fracture and all are likely to produce severe pain and possibly immobility, shock, nausea and vomiting: compression fracture, burst fracture and spinal dislocation. There may be signs of swelling, bruising and internal bleeding. In all cases of accidental injury involving the back, it is essential to call for emergency medical help and not to move the patient in any way, except if there is immediate danger to life. A spinal fracture can be highly unstable and there is a risk of permanent damage to the spinal cord and paralysis.

Compression fracture: A compression fracture is one in which the vertebra collapses, having first become weakened by the development of a series of small cracks through the body of the vertebra. The usual cause is osteoporosis. In the osteoporotic spine, there may be a series of such collapses resulting in a general loss of height. Treatment comprises analgesic medication and either vertebroplasty or kyphoplasty (*see* page 164).

Burst fracture: A burst fracture, which is most likely to occur following trauma, involves shattering or crushing of the vertebra(e) with the production of shards or free fragments of bone. This is an extremely painful injury posing a high risk of damage to the spinal cord. The patient must be immobilized before being moved and requires immediate pain relief. Once admitted to hospital, x-rays and other scans and investigations are likely to be carried out to determine the precise nature of the injury. Treatment depends upon the outcome of this but may involve surgery (spinal fusion) or immobilization with a body cast or back brace for up to 3 months.

In a fracture with dislocation there is the additional factor of joint surfaces being displaced. Treatment is essentially the same as for a burst fracture, with surgery likely to be required.

Spinal dislocation

Spinal dislocation describes an injury in which one or more joints between vertebrae have been forced out of place. If *total*, there is no longer any contact between the surfaces that are normally articulated. In a *partial* dislocation or *subluxation*, some degree of contact remains. Spinal dislocation is nearly always caused by a traumatic accident and is usually accompanied by fracture. Symptoms are essentially the same as for fracture but with noticeable deformity and visible swelling often present. Once again, this type of injury constitutes an emergency requiring skilled, professional care and above all, immobilization of the patient before he or she can be moved. Following investigation and evaluation in hospital, treatment is likely to comprise surgical spinal fusion and manipulation to realign the spine. Immobilization and traction may be needed as part of ongoing treatment. Recovery can be prolonged. The cervical spine is the most susceptible to dislocation but dislocation in the thoracic spine is the cause of 80% of all cases of paraplegia (paralysis of the legs, often involving loss of control of the bladder and bowel).

11. Childhood Back Pain

Back pain is fairly common among children and adolescents and, as is the case in adults, much of it arises as a result of poor posture and subjecting the spine to stresses and strains through inappropriate activity. In other children it may be attributed to 'growing pains' or a disparity between the rates of growth in different areas of the skeleton and musculature. However, in some cases, back pain is a sign of an underlying condition or disorder and any symptoms in a child warrant medical evaluation, investigation and monitoring.

Childhood spondylolisthesis

In children, spondylolisthesis arises due to an inherent weakness or defect in the bony neural arch between the paired articular processes of two adjacent, lumbar vertebrae. Loading pressure on the spine may cause cracking in the weakened bone with a slight forward movement of the upper vertebra relative to the one beneath it. Symptoms include pain and stiffness and this may be treated with analgesic medication and, probably, modification and reduction of movement and activity. The condition requires ongoing monitoring and may need corrective surgery in the form of *vertebral spinal fusion* if it progresses beyond a certain point.

Compressive stress fracture of the pars interarticularis

The pars interarticularis is the portion of bone located between the superior and inferior articular processes of a vertebra on either side. In young athletes whose sport involves a lot of backward bending and rotation of the spine, such as tennis, cricket (fast bowling) and baseball, an overuse or repetitive stress fracture may occur in the pars interarticularis of a lumbar vertebra. This usually occurs on one side only but may affect both sides of the vertebra and most commonly it is L4 or L5 that is involved. If on one side only, the fracture normally occurs on the opposite side to that of the repetitive activity. Hence in a right-handed bowler, the injury occurs on the left side of the vertebra. Symptoms include pain on the affected side(s) and this is exacerbated with extension and backwards bending. Pain may arise suddenly or gradually and is accompanied by tenderness when the affected area is pressed externally. The *hamstring* and *gluteal* muscles are sometimes bunched and tight. A young sportsperson exhibiting these symptoms should undergo medical investigation, as it is not uncommon for this injury to go undetected at first. As with all injuries, a prompt diagnosis offers the best chance of an early recovery. Investigation may involve x-rays and/or an MRI scan.

Treatment includes giving analgesic pain relief and complete rest from the sport that caused the injury. Physiotherapy and rehabilitation exercises, with reduced or modified activity for 6 months are likely to be needed. If the sport is resumed, training to alter the way the activity is performed is advisable to prevent recurrence. One-sided fractures usually heal completely with those at the L4 level being less problematic than those at L5. Recovery from a fracture on both sides tends to be more complicated and carries a risk of the future development of spondylolisthesis.

Scheuermann's disease/kyphosis

This is a disorder of the spine belonging to a group of conditions known collectively as the *osteochondroses*. It is a developmental disorder that generally presents during adolescence and it is more common in boys than in girls. About 8% of all children have this disorder and it affects the thoracic spine, generally between the level of T7 to T9. The most notable feature is a rounded or hunched back (kyphosis) together with a forward bending profile. It is caused by irregular, differential rates of growth between the front and back portions of affected vertebrae. This leads to the development of an abnormal wedge shape in the body of the vertebra(e) instead of the usual rounded appearance and it is this which produces the kyphosis. The wedge shape is readily apparent on x-rays of the spine. This disorder tends to cause discomfort rather than severe pain and indeed, many children are entirely pain free. The cause is unknown but infection, accidental injury and poor circulation during phases of rapid growth may be among implicated factors.

Treatment is variable depending upon the nature and severity of symptoms. Monitoring may be all that is needed in some cases but in others, physiotherapy and spinal strengthening exercises, along with mild analgesic medication, may be required. It may be recommended that the child wear a back brace but unfortunately, this is highly unpopular among the age group concerned and various psychological issues may need to be addressed. Support in the form of psychological counselling may prove helpful, along with explaining the nature of the disorder to the child's friends and peer group to lessen the risk of teasing or bullying. Surgery (in the form of spinal fusion) is rarely needed and would only be considered in cases of extreme and progressive curvature or where there is severe pain or neurological damage. In later life the deformity can be a focus for arthritis and it is at this point that pain may become a greater problem, necessitating other forms of treatment, including taking analgesic and anti-inflammatory medication.

Achondroplasia

Achondroplasia is the most common form of abnormally short stature (dwarfism). It is an autosomal, dominant genetic disorder and this means that a mutation in only one copy of the responsible gene inherited from each parent is needed for the condition to be manifested. In 75% of all cases, the mutation in the gene has been spontaneous, arising for an unknown reason in that particular child who is born to parents of normal stature. In the remainder of cases the condition is inherited. The responsible gene, designated FGF3, codes information for fibroplast growth factor receptors number 3. Growth factors are natural biochemicals responsible for growth and to work, they must first bind to the surface of special receptors designed to receive them. In acondroplasia the mutation in FGF3 prevents this from happening and the areas that are affected are cartilage and the central nervous system.

The disorder prevents cartilage from turning into bone so that normal growth is restricted. There is extreme shortening of the thigh bones and upper arm bones and shortened hands and feet, with abnormal spacing between the 3rd and 4th digits. The pelvis is squared with a small sacrosciatic notch and the *pedicles* of the vertebrae are also shortened. There is a characteristic chevron shape in the epiphyses (the specialized plates of cartilage at the head of the long bones in children that are vitally important for growth). There is restricted growth at the base of the skull and the head may appear large, with a flat nose and large forehead. In some children, teeth are overcrowded leading to dental problems. Bowed legs and ear infections are common among affected infants and in some children, there is kyphosis in the region of the junction between the thoracic and lumbar spine. There is a risk of hydrocephalus (an abnormal collection of cerebrospinal fluid within the skull), compression of the spinal cord and breathing difficulties among severely affected children. The torso is of normal size and affected adults reach a height of about 4 feet.

Children with achondroplasia tend to reach physical developmental milestones later than the norm but there is no intellectual impairment.

There is no cure for achondroplasia and any treatment given is aimed at relieving any problematic symptoms that may be present to a greater or lesser degree. But affected children may be given growth hormone to stimulate bone development. Surgery may be needed to correct spinal problems and to relieve compression of the cord. If present, hydrocephalus always necessitates treatment to drain fluid. There may be considerable psychosocial problems as the child grows and becomes more aware and so specialist counselling and support services can be needed. In adult life, a common complication of the condition is lumbar/sacral spinal stenosis and this is likely to require corrective surgery.

Still's disease or juvenile rheumatoid arthritis/JRA

Still's disease is a particular type of juvenile rheumatoid arthritis that is also known as *systemic-onset JRA*. It accounts for about a fifth of all cases of JRA arising in children. Symptoms may occur gradually or develop rapidly and they number pain and inflammation in both small and large joints, including those of the spine. Often this begins in the fingers and then spreads to other joints in a characteristic symmetrical fashion – wrists, elbows, knees and ankles. Sometimes only one joint is involved. Accompanying the arthritis there may be fever, skin rash, eye inflammation, blood changes and an enlargement of glands, including the spleen. There may be a stiff, painful neck, muscle wastage, disrupted growth and a receded chin. These symptoms may precede the typical arthritic signs in some children. There may be active phases of the disease punctuated with interludes of remission. Treatment involves drug therapy, such as the use of non-steroidal, anti-inflammatory medication and gold salts, and bed-rest with modified activity. Some affected children may go on to develop ankylosing spondylitis.

Sacral agenesis/hyperplasia of the sacrum

A rare, congenital deformity of the sacrum which arises early on during the 4th to 6th week of foetal development. The malformation can present in different ways including absence of the sacrum or as a one-sided or bilateral deformity. This abnormality is normally detected before birth by means of foetal scanning. Children born with this condition may have severe disabilities with instability of the lower spine and pelvis, scoliosis, hip displacement and lower leg deformities. There may be partial or total incontinence. Treatment is aimed at relieving the effects of these problems and helping the child to enjoy the best possible quality of life. There is a need for continued support and therapy of various kinds, both for the child and for the family involved.

12. Other (Rare) Diseases and Conditions that May Be Associated with Back Pain

Spinal tumours

A tumour is an abnormal mass in any part of the body caused by an unusual growth of tissue and sometimes, a rapid, uncontrolled multiplication of calls. A tumour may be *benign* (non-cancerous) or *malignant* (cancerous). A malignant tumour is one that usually proliferates rapidly and destroys surrounding healthy tissue. It can spread (*metastasize*) by seeding cells into the blood and lymphatic system and these may then travel to lodge elsewhere in the body and grow into new *metastases* (cancer). Tumours tend to be classified according to the tissue type of which they are composed, eg myoma (largely muscle fibres). Cancerous tumours are also defined as either *primary* or *secondary*. A primary tumour is one that originates within the tissues in which it is found. A secondary tumour is another name for a metastasis, being a malignant tumour that has metastasized from a primary cancer in another area.

Spinal tumours can grow in any area of the spine and affect a variety of the tissues and structures that are present. They are, however, rare with an incidence in the UK of around 750 new cases each year. Most cancerous tumours of the spine are secondary in nature. In women, the site of the primary tumour is usually the breast or lung; in men, it is commonly the prostate gland or lung. Both benign and cancerous spinal tumours can cause serious symptoms with pain being present in 80% of all cases. However, the nature and severity of this depends upon the location and rate of growth of the mass. These tumours grow in or around the structures associated with the vertebrae, hence compression of the spinal cord or nerve roots is frequently present, producing symptoms of weakness, numbness, tingling in the limbs or even degrees of paralysis, in severe cases.

Benign tumours

Aneurysmal bone cyst or ABC: Strictly speaking an ABC is a type of cyst rather than a tumour and if found in the back, it usually occurs in the lumbar spine. It produces acute pain that comes on suddenly and worsens over a period of 2 to 3 months with reddening, swelling and heating of the skin over the affected area. If it arises in the cervical spine or skull, there may be headaches. An ABC can arise in any person but young women are at greater risk. The cause is unknown but there may be a link with previous injury or another type of tumour in some cases. Surgery to remove the cyst is the preferred method of treatment, provided that the growth is in an accessible place.

Giant cell tumour or GCT: This type of tumour mainly occurs in young adults, especially women and as the name suggests, characteristically features cells of abnormally large proportions. It causes pain and this increases as the tumour grows and if a joint is involved, there may be swelling, tenderness and restriction of associated movement. Treatment is by means of surgery to remove the mass and/or radiotherapy. There is a slight risk that a GCT may become cancerous if left untreated.

Hemangioma: This type of tumour is most commonly found in the lumbar or thoracic spine and it is most prevalent in middle-aged women. It is sometimes likened to an internal birthmark and it often produces no symptoms and can be safely left alone. Rarely, there may be bleeding into the spinal canal and pressure on the spinal cord or nerve roots, causing pain and other symptoms that then require treatment.

Ostoid osteoma: This is a tumour that usually arises in the lumbar spine but may occur elsewhere. It produces an aching pain that is worse at night and it is usually managed with analgesic medication. Rarely, the tumour may cause spinal deformity and if it arises in the *epiphysis* of a long bone in a child, it may cause interference with growth. However, those most at risk are young men between the ages of 20 and 40 years.

Malignant tumours
Osteoblastoma: This is a rare type of tumour that is most commonly found in the lumbar spine and is usually malignant but may sometimes be benign. It usually affects young males aged 20 to 30 years.

Chondrosarcoma: This is a cancer of immature or fully formed cartilaginous cells that usually arises in the pelvic girdle, lumbar or thoracic spine or in long bones. It is slow growing and causes localized pain at the site of the mass and sometimes, numbness or weakness in a (lower) limb and abnormal reflexes. It is a tumour that may be difficult to treat surgically and it most commonly affects middle-aged men over the age of 40 years.

Chordoma: This rare, slow-growing tumour is most usually found in the sacral spine or at the base of the skull. There is pain of varying degrees of intensity and there may be symptoms of spinal cord or nerve root compression. If occurring in the sacral area, the tumour may produce a notable mass and this can sometimes interfere with bladder and bowel function. Headaches and blurred vision may occur if the tumour is located at the top of the spine or base of the skull. Surgery, when possible, is the preferred form of treatment.

Osteosarcoma: This is a type of bone cancer that is usually found in the long bones. It rarely affects the spine but if present, causes symptoms of pain, neurological effects such as loss of sensation, numbness, weakness, tingling and degrees of paralysis. There may possibly be a loss of height due to increased occurrence of *fractures*. This tumour most commonly affects young men and treatment methods include *surgery*, radiotherapy and chemotherapy.

Lymphoma: This is a cancer of the lymphatic system and one that may arise at multiple sites in the spine. It causes pain and symptoms of spinal cord compression including weakness, numbness, tingling, loss of reflexes and degrees of paralysis. Lymph nodes become enlarged and there may be fever, anaemia and weight loss. Treatment methods include surgery, radiotherapy and chemotherapy and the prognosis is best when the disease is detected at an early stage. Lymphoma most commonly affects middle-aged adults between the ages of 40 and 60 years.

Multiple myeloma: This is the most common type of *round cell tumour* involving bone marrow cells. It causes destruction of bone tissue, deformities and increased likelihood of fractures. If present in the spine it usually arises at multiple sites. There is pain that increases with movement and is persistent if a fracture is present. It most commonly affects older adults aged between 50 and 80 years and it is treated by means of radiotherapy and chemotherapy.

Plasmacytoma: This is a type of round cell tumour involving plasma cells and arising either at a single or multiple sites in the spine, generally in the thoracic and lumbar regions. There is a reduction in all other types of blood cells, both white and red and possible symptoms include tiredness, anaemia and an increased likelihood of opportunistic infections. It is most likely to affect men aged over 50 years and it is treated by means of radiotherapy and chemotherapy.

Ewing's sarcoma: This is a highly malignant but rare form of bone cancer, most commonly affecting children and young adults. Males are at greater risk and this bone cancer occurs at a younger age than any other form of the disease, with a peak incidence between the ages of 10 and 20 years. It usually first arises in the limb or pelvic bones but is liable to soon spread to other parts of the body. Symptoms include a high temperature and a raised white blood cell count, weight loss and anorexia. Also, there may be sensations of tingling, numbness and weakness and sometimes paralysis. It is treated by means of radiotherapy and chemotherapy and surgical amputation of a limb may be required in some cases. Combined therapy produces a cure in over 60% of young people with localized disease, with early detection offering the best chance of success.

Paget's disease of bone or osteitis deformans

This is a chronic disease that particularly affects the long bones, spine and skull and causes the bones to become thickened, soft and weak with a disorganized structure. It most commonly affects adults, particularly men, aged over 40 years. Symptoms include pain in the bones and this is of an aching nature and may be severe, especially at night. The skull may become enlarged, nerves compressed and damaged, especially in the spine and possibly causing degrees of paralysis. There may be bowing of the spine and legs and the bones are liable to fracture. Headaches and loss of hearing are other possible symptoms. The signs may be vague or absent in the early stages of the disease and it tends to progress in active phases interspersed with periods of quiescence.

There is no cure and treatment is symptomatic, aimed at relief of pain and management. Various drugs may be used, including salicylates, non-steroidal anti-inflammatory medication, calcitonin and biphosphonates. Orthopaedic surgery and mobility aids may be needed. Heat in the form of heat pads and hot baths are helpful, as is bed-rest during acute attacks. The cause is unknown but there is a greater risk for individuals with a family member already affected. Various complications can occur, including compression of the brain due to skull enlargement, hypertension and heart disease. Paget's disease is sometimes misdiagnosed as secondary bone cancer (especially in those previously treated for primary breast or prostate gland cancer), or in patients who have an overactive parathyroid gland.

Kidney stones or calculi

Kidney stones comprise deposits of hard material, varying in size, that may form and collect within the kidneys and pass into the *ureters*, (the tubes through which urine passes from the bladder to the outside). The stones are composed of various substances, including calcium phosphate, calcium oxalate, ammonium phosphate, calcium carbonate and uric acid or urates. Kidney stones most commonly affect adults aged over 30 years, with men being at slightly higher risk. A sedentary life style is a further predisposing factor. Symptoms include a sharp, severe and intermittent stabbing pain in the back and small amounts of blood may be present in the urine (*haematuria*). A person with symptoms of kidney stones should seek medical advice and treatment depends upon the size and nature of the calculi. If they are small (*gravel*) they may be passed spontaneously with the flow of urine. However, larger stones may require treatment with ultrasound in order to break them up so that they can be passed naturally or, if this is unsuccessful or cannot be used, surgical removal may be needed.

A person with kidney stones should drink plenty of fluids to help flush the system. The stones may have formed due to a change in the acidity or alkalinity of the urine hence medication to alter this may be required. If the stones are mainly composed of calcium then bendrofluazide may be prescribed. Dietary changes to avoid foods containing high levels of calcium and/or phosphorus may be advised. Various factors favour the formation of kidney stones, including a high level of calcium in urine (*hypercalcuria*), changes in acidity or alkalinity of urine, changes in concentration of urine, which may arise if too little fluid is drunk and /or with excessive sweating. Also, gout (deposits of uric acid), familial tendency, a diet deficient in vitamin A and an overactive parathyroid gland are further risk factors.

Polycystic kidney disease or PKD

PKD is one of a group of abnormal, inherited disorders of the kidneys characterized by the development of cysts. The disorders may be either dominant or recessive in their pattern of inheritance. Different types of these disorders may be present before birth or arise in childhood or adult life. The kidneys enlarge and have a reduced ability to perform their natural function of cleansing the blood and excreting urine. In this disease, healthy kidney tissue is gradually replaced by cysts and these are composed of abnormal, expanded portions of kidney tubules. The cysts may cause low back pain or sharp pain of a colicky nature in the back. Also, there may be blood in the urine, high blood pressure and, in rare cases, a life-threatening aneurysm or sub-arachnoid haemorrhage (a type of bleeding in the brain). Treatment depends upon the severity of symptoms and the stage of the disease and it is aimed at preserving kidney function, treating any infections and managing high blood pressure. Dialysis and/or a kidney transplant may eventually be needed. The cause of PKD is usually a mutant gene located on chromosome 16 and the condition reduces natural life expectancy. People with a family history of the disorder should receive genetic counselling.

Pancreatic cancer

Pancreatic cancer is an abnormal, malignant proliferation of cells within the pancreas and most commonly affects middle-aged adults with men being at somewhat greater risk. The pancreas is a vital gland located between the duodenum and the spleen and it produces the hormone insulin and digestive enzymes. In the early stages there may be few symptoms but those that do occur include abdominal pain radiating into the back that lessens with forward bending, weight loss, gastrointestinal bleeding, jaundice and severe skin itching. Treatment methods include chemotherapy, radiotherapy and possibly surgery, analgesic medication, injections of pancreatic enzymes and possibly insulin and anti-itching preparations. Risk factors for this type of cancer include pancreatitis (inflammation of the pancreas), diabetes, smoking and alcohol abuse. It is incurable and treatment is palliative, to relieve symptoms and enhance quality of life.

Endometriosis

Endometriosis is a condition that affects women of childbearing age in which cells from the *endometrium* (the lining of the womb) become lodged elsewhere in the body, usually in the *fallopian tubes, ovaries* or muscular wall of the womb. Symptoms include pelvic and low back pain that is persistent and usually worse during menstruation. Heavy period bleeding and pain during intercourse are common. Treatment methods include oral hormone supplements and surgery. The cause is unknown but it poses a risk of the formation of pelvic cysts and infertility.

Rheumatoid arthritis

Rheumatoid arthritis is the second most common form of disease of the joints and it usually affects the feet, ankles, fingers and wrists but can involve the spine. Diagnosis is made by means of x-rays and these reveal a typical pattern of changes around the inflamed joint, known as *rheumatoid erosions*. At first there is swelling of the joint and inflammation of the *synovial membrane* (the membranous sac surrounding the joint), followed by erosion and loss of cartilage and bone. A blood test reveals the presence of *serum rheumatoid factor antibody* the presence of which is characteristic. All age groups are affected, especially those aged between 30 and 50 years, with women at higher risk. Symptoms usually arise slowly and insidiously but occasionally may be rapid in onset. There is inflammation, tenderness and pain in the affected joints and stiffness that is worse on first arising in the morning. Later in the day, the person may feel general tiredness and malaise. Deformity in affected joints is likely to arise. In some people, an active phase is followed by a long period of remission. Rest in bed during active phases is recommended and adequate rest and good nutrition is essential at all times. Drugs used in treatment include aspirin and salicylates, nonsteroidal anti-inflammatory preparations and slow-acting agents such as penicillamine, sulphasalazine, gold and hydrochloroquine. Many patients improve with treatment and the condition varies greatly in severity. At its worst it is progressively and severely disabling but others less severely affected are able to lead a relatively normal life. The cause is unknown but appears to involve several genetic factors and most of those affected have a particular antibody, designated HLA-DR4.

Osteomyelitis

Osteomyelitis is inflammation and infection of bone marrow and bones and it may exist in acute and chronic form. It affects people of all ages but in children is more likely to arise between the ages of 5 to 14 years. The infection may be general or localized; in children it usually affects the long bones and in adults, the spine and pelvis. Symptoms include worsening pain in the affected bone, swelling, fever, muscle spasm, redness and heat in the skin over the area involved. Treatment may necessitate hospital admission for high doses of antibiotics, possibly given intravenously. Bed-rest is needed until the infection has cleared and symptoms have subsided. Analgesic medication is likely to be required and antibiotic treatment may last for several weeks. The infection is usually caused by staphylococcal bacteria entering the bloodstream following an infection elsewhere such as from a boil, or after injury or surgery. Sometimes an acute attack can be followed by the development of a chronic condition, with periodic flare-ups. This may be due to bits of debris and dead bone (or *sequestra*) that have been left behind, perhaps after injury, providing a focus for irritation and infection.

Osteomalacia

Osteomalacia is a softening of bones and the adult equivalent of rickets in children, caused by a lack of vitamin D. This vitamin is obtained from the diet and is also produced when the skin is exposed to the sun and it is necessary for the absorption of dietary calcium. The condition is most likely to affect the elderly but also others who have a low intake of calcium combined with little sun exposure. Asian women who cover up completely for religious reasons may be at greater risk, especially if their diet is low in calcium-containing foods. Treatment methods include dietary modification and supplements of necessary minerals and bone-strengthening preparations such as biphosphonates.

Ulcerative colitis

Ulcerative colitis is inflammation of the colon with possible development of ulcers and it is a severe, chronic disorder and one that tends to recur. It is most prevalent in young adults, especially women, between the ages of 16 to 45 years. The usual symptoms include abdominal pain, watery diarrhoea containing blood, anaemia, fever, weight loss and sweating. However, there can also be a connection with inflammation of the sacroiliac joint and low back pain. Treatment is by means of bed-rest and various drugs, including corticosteroids, sulphasalazine and azathioprine, along with iron supplements and a low roughage diet. In rare cases, there can be life-threatening complications but most patients respond well to treatment. The cause is unknown but there may be a genetic/-familial susceptibility and risks increase with excess consumption of alcohol. Also, people with this condition are at greater risk of contracting cancer of the colon.

Crohn's disease

Crohn's disease causes inflammation of the lower part of the small intestine, leading to ulceration and thickening. It most commonly affects young adults aged between 20 and 40 years and tends to recur. The usual symptoms are spasmodic abdominal pains, slight fever, nausea, loss of weight and lack of appetite, diarrhoea and abdominal distension. There is a thickening of the ileum that can sometimes be felt externally. However, there can also be a connection with inflammation of the sacroiliac joint and low back pain. Treatment consists of rest and eating a low-fibre diet that is high in vitamins. Analgesic drugs and vitamin supplements may be prescribed and also antibiotics and corticosteroids. Occasionally, if there is a complete blockage or failure to respond to medical treatment, admittance to hospital for surgical removal of the affected part may be necessary. The cause is unknown although there may be a tendency for Crohn's disease to occur in families and hence a genetic link. People with food allergies are more susceptible and the disease carries an increased risk of cancer of the intestine.

Reiter's syndrome (RS)

RS is a disease that produces symptoms of urethritis, conjunctivitis and reactive arthritis, affecting joints including those of the spine, resulting from infection elsewhere. This disease most commonly affects young males aged between 12 and 40 years. Early symptoms include fever, frequent urination and infected discharge, inflamed, watering eyes, pains in affected joints and reddened skin. Mouth ulcers may develop. Treatment involves antibiotics and analgesic drugs, with physiotherapy and exercises for affected joints. There are two forms of RS and one of these is thought to be sexually transmitted, while the other results from infection in the gastrointestinal tract (dysenteric RS). Women, children and the elderly are usually affected by the dysenteric form, which is less common and is believed to have a genetic tendency for its occurrence.

Psoriasis

Psoriasis is a chronic skin disorder that tends to remain throughout life and is characterized by alternating active and quiescent periods. In some people it is associated with a severe and disabling form of arthritis affecting the joints, including those of the spine. The condition usually arises in adolescence or early adulthood with the appearance of red, roughened skin patches covered by shiny, silvery scales. Some of those affected develop a more extreme skin reaction known as exfoliative psoriatic dermatitis in which there is severe thickening and a deterioration in general health. Patients with this form of the disease and those with psoriatic arthritis may require hospital treatment with methotrexate (a potent, anti-metabolite preparation). The cause is not known but there is often a familial tendency and white-skinned people are far more likely to be affected than those of African-Caribbean or Asian origin.

Shingles

Shingles is an infection produced by the *Varicella-zoster* virus that is also the cause of chickenpox in children. The infection affects the central nervous system, more specifically the spinal cord (dorsal root ganglia) and it follows the course of a nerve, producing severe pain and small, yellow blisters on the skin. Adults of all ages may be affected but particularly those aged over 50 years. Those most at risk are people who are generally somewhat ill or 'run-down', perhaps following illness or treatment with immunosuppressive drugs or after a period of stress; also, those with Hodgkin's disease. Symptoms include pain, sometimes severe and this may be in the back or chest and it can persist for some time (post-herpetic neuralgia). Blisters appear on the skin following the route of the nerve, often in a semi-circular pattern on the chest, side and back. Pain-relieving drugs, corticosteroids and antivirals such as acyclovir may be prescribed and warm compresses and application of heat can also prove soothing. Although it may take some weeks, most people recover fully and they are then likely to have immunity from future attacks of the illness.

Seronegative spondyloarthropathy

This is a collective name for a group of disorders affecting the *axial skeleton* (skull, vertebral column, ribs and sternum) and their associated joints and also, peripheral joints. There is accompanying inflammation at the sites of insertion of tendons and ligaments to bone (*enthesitis*). These disorders are characterized by a high incidence of human leucocyte antigen HLA-B27 but an absence of rheumatoid factor. Typical symptoms include back pain, stiffness on first arising in the morning, chest pain (pleurisy), restricted movement, pain in hips, knees and shoulders, tiredness, weight loss, fever and, possibly, heart murmur. Among this group of disorders are: Reiter's syndrome, JRA, inflammatory bowel diseases (Crohn's and ulcerative colitis), ankylosing spondylitis, psoriatic arthritis and reactive arthritis.

Gout

Gout is a disorder caused by an imbalance of uric acid (an organic acid containing nitrogen, being the end product of protein metabolism) in the body. It leads to deposition of this substance as salts (*urates*) of the acid in the joints, possibly including those of the spine, causing inflammation and pain. Older adults are most likely to be affected, particularly men aged over 60 years. Gout is uncommon in people aged below 40 years unless there is family history of the disorder. Symptoms include inflammation, swelling, reddening, tenderness and severe pain in affected joints (gouty arthritis). Deposits of the salts (called *tophi*) may reach the stage where they prohibit further use of the joints, causing hands and feet to become 'set' in a particular position. Treatment for an acute attack is usually colchicines, a preparation that relieves pain and inflammation and has been used (as *colchium*) for many centuries. Prevention of further attacks is by means of drugs that increase the excretion of waste salts or slow their formation and also analgesic and non-steroidal anti-inflammatory preparations. Rest to keep weight off the affected joints is recommended until symptoms subside. Certain drugs and antibiotics increase the risk of developing gout as do some blood diseases such as leukaemia. In addition, there is often a familial, genetic predisposition involved.

13. Medical Consultations and Investigations – What to Expect

The GP

If back pain is severe or recurrent, or if it has persisted for sometime without any noticeable improvement, or if it is getting worse, it is natural to seek medical help. Almost universally in the UK, the first port of call for the majority of people is their family doctor or general practitioner (GP). As mentioned above, GPs have been advised to adopt a 'triage' approach when dealing with a patient complaining of back pain. This means that the doctor will hope to be able to assign the patient to one of three categories: simple back pain; back pain with nerve root symptoms; other potentially more serious, underlying pathology (*see also* page 21).

In order to assign the patient to one of these groups and to arrive at a clearer understanding of the nature of the problem, the doctor will wish to obtain as much information as possible. A vital part of this is listening to, and noting, the patient's account of his or her experience and asking questions to clarify details. Questions that may be asked are likely to include: when and how did the pain begin, was it related to any particular incident or physical activity and what is the nature and severity of the pain?

An assessment of the patient's state of health and a physical examination is likely to be carried out and this will probably necessitate the removal of outer clothing. While standing, the patient may be asked to bend the back in each direction, forwards, backwards and sideways, in order to assess the degree of flexibility of the spine. The doctor will wish to know which, if any, of these movements make the pain worse. In the event of signs of nerve root involvement, limb reflexes and muscle strength will be tested with the patient lying down. While still lying on the bed, the patient may be asked to raise each leg in turn and the doctor may gently palpate the lower back and hip joints.

Throughout the whole consultation, the doctor will be on the lookout for *red flag* and *yellow flag* signs. Red flags, eg sudden, unexplained weight loss, gastrointestinal disturbance and other physiological symptoms, are indications of potentially serious disorders. Neurological symptoms, eg interference with, or loss of control of, the bladder or bowel, also necessitate prompt investigation.

Yellow flags cover the psychological aspects of back pain. These include anticipatory fear of pain with movement. This is a fear that the pain itself is harmful and that its occurrence worsens the back problem – known as *fear avoidance* behaviour. Also included are anxiety and stress – perhaps related to the perceived ability to work or to function as before in pursuing sporting activities or normal social interactions. It is common for negative thinking to arise in relation to back pain, especially when the pain is felt to be severe and disabling. In extreme cases, the person may adopt an entirely pessimistic attitude and start to believe in a worst-case scenario such as becoming paralysed, wheelchair bound or succumbing to spinal cancer. In psychology, these are called 'catastrophic thoughts' and the mental process that gives rise to them is termed 'catastrophizing'. It is important to recognize their presence and significance since it has been proved that they interfere considerably with recovery and greatly increase the risk of back pain becoming chronic.

In fact, it has been shown that yellow flags are the strongest early predictors of chronicity, over and above the actual severity of the problem in the person's back. There is a higher risk of the development of depression with any chronic pain condition and back pain is no exception to this rule. Also, a patient who is already suffering with depression or any other anxiety-related disorder runs a far higher risk of developing chronic back pain.

For all these reasons the GP will note yellow flag signs and will certainly take them seriously. Help with these may even be of greater importance at this stage than treatment for the actual pain in the back.

In most instances, the judgement made by the GP will be to assign the patient to the simple back pain category. Even when the pain is severe, the patient can be reassured that this will ease with time and the likely recommendation will be to take over-the-counter medication, such as paracetamol or ibuprofen, for the pain. The patient may be referred to the practice physiotherapist and/or be given an exercise sheet and general advice about returning to normal levels of activity. However, the doctor may sometimes prescribe medication, such as a codeine-based preparation (a stronger painkiller) or a muscle-relaxant (diazepam), or take a blood sample for laboratory analysis.

If red flags are present or suspected, the patient will have a prompt referral for further investigations to be carried out but the speed of this very much depends upon the patient's condition and the degree of urgency. In the rarest cases there might be immediate referral to hospital but a more likely situation would be a 'fast-track' appointment to see an appropriate specialist. This would also apply if the patient is found to have severe nerve root pain and in this case strong analgesic and anti-inflammatory medication is likely to be prescribed immediately. The referral may be to an orthopaedic or musculo-skeletal consultant, a multi-disciplinary pain team or to some other specialist, depending upon the judgement that has been made by the GP and the nature of the services provided by the local health authority.

In the UK, there is a blurring of the boundaries between primary care provided by GPs and specialist services as the latter may be either hospital or community-based or a combination of both. A recent survey has shown that there is wide variation in the way services are organized in different health authorities and in one sense this does not matter. The only important factor is that patients with severe and/or chronic back pain receive help and appropriate care and treatment according to their needs.

Seeing the specialist

In the majority of cases, by the time a back-pain patient gets to see a specialist he or she has had a problem that has persisted for some time. It is likely that various treatments have already been tried and have failed to provide any lasting solution but only some amelioration of the pain. By this point, most patients find themselves having to take sometimes quite high doses of (strong) analgesics in order to function and to get through the day. The level of pain and interference with normal life is possibly severe and the situation may have worsened with the passage of time.

The specialist or consultant will have received notes about the patient's medical history in advance of the appointment. These will not only include details about the current back pain problem but also any other information that might be relevant, such as an existing condition or disorder or the presence of yellow flag signs. Reading the notes enables the specialist to gain insight and perhaps form some opinion about the possible nature of the problem. However, the specialist will naturally wish to conduct a detailed and thorough examination of the patient and for this reason a first consultation usually lasts for about half an hour.

During the opening discussion, the patient will be asked to describe the problem and will be encouraged to talk about any concerns and fears that may be present. A physical examination normally follows and for this the patient is asked to remove outer clothing. The specialist will wish to ascertain the degree of movement and the flexibility of the spine and limbs and to test reflexes and to discover which movements exacerbate the pain. The specialist will use palpatory skills to discover signs of disorder and dysfunction in the pelvis, spine and related soft tissues. This involves using physical touch and gentle pressure to detect from the outside subtle changes that are taking place or have taken place within. Any symptoms relating to nerve root or spinal cord pressure, such as a loss of muscle tone and weakness or impairment of bladder or bowel control, will also be assessed.

When the patient is once more dressed, the consultation will end with a discussion on the possible nature of the problem and what the solution may be, as well as reassurance for the patient about any steps that may prove necessary. The consultant may not give a definitive diagnosis at this stage but may wish to refer the patient for some form of scan or other investigation. However, it is likely that possible treatment options will be raised to be finally decided upon later during a follow-up consultation, once the results of any investigations are available.

Investigative techniques

Blood tests

Blood tests may be carried out for a variety of reasons as part of the investigation into a possible cause for the back pain but particularly to provide evidence of the possible existence of some underlying disease or condition that might be responsible. Blood tests carried out to look for disorders of the spine include ESR (Erythrocyte [red blood cell] Sedimentation Rate), full blood count, vitamin D assay, plasma viscosity, alkaline phosphatase enzyme test, electrophoretic strip (testing the level of plasma protein), rheumatoid factor tests, prostate specific antigen test and acid phosphatase test (for disorders of the male prostate gland) and uric acid levels (for presence of gout). Disorders implicated in back pain that may be highlighted by blood tests include inflammatory diseases, such as gout, ankylosing spondylitis, rheumatoid arthritis, spondyloarthropathy, Crohn's disease and ulcerative colitis, as well as other diseases such as cancer. However, it should be borne in mind that a request to provide a blood sample is a fairly routine occurrence and it should not in any way be viewed as a cause for anxiety or concern.

X-rays

In the past, any person suffering from persistent back pain would almost certainly have had x-ray images taken of the spine in an effort to identify the cause of the problem. But in modern medicine, plain x-rays are far less likely to be called for and for very sound reasons. Firstly, x-rays can only show a two-dimensional view of the bones themselves and the spaces between them, and they are very much a blunt instrument when it comes to pinpointing the likely cause of pain. Also, as has been mentioned previously, x-rays commonly reveal exactly the same kind of degenerative and structural changes in the spines of people who are pain free as in those who are suffering from back pain. Where x-rays do come into their own and are of fundamental importance is in those patients suspected of having sustained a spinal fracture. This might be a compression fracture in an elderly patient or a younger person who has sustained an accidental traumatic injury to the back. A further use for x-rays in back pain is to guide certain forms of treatment such as epidural steroid injections (fluoroscopy) and provocation discography.

Magnetic Resonance Imaging or MRI scan

An MRI scanner uses a powerful magnetic field combined with radio waves to generate images of structures within the body. Hydrogen atoms that form part of water molecules contained within the tissue being scanned are induced by means of magnets to alter their position, emitting minute radio signals in the process, and these are detected by a receiver built into the machine. The strength of the signals varies according to the type and nature of the tissue being scanned. A computer within the machine is able to interpret the signals and use them to generate images of the scanned tissue. Although each of these is produced as a two-dimensional 'slice', they can be taken in series and from different angles to create a three-dimensional picture, with the images obtained being viewed on a computer screen. MRI is excellent for producing images of soft tissues such as ligaments, cartilage, nerves, muscles and blood vessels, disc prolapses and bulges, and areas of inflammation and swelling. It is not useful for looking at bones or for detecting alterations and changes that may have taken place within them.

To undergo the scan, the patient must lie on a motorized bed and this is then positioned within a large, open-ended cylinder. The person has a small receiving device placed around the area being scanned and must lie very still for the duration of the process. The machine is operated remotely by a radiographer who is stationed in an adjacent room. The radiographer can see what is happening through a glass window and communication is maintained by means of an intercom. The scanner makes quite a lot of noise due to the movement of magnets within it and some people find the process quite trying and difficult to endure. The problems lie with the necessity to remain very still and also, for some, a feeling of claustrophobia.

A typical scan lasts for about 20 to 30 minutes. It is an outpatient procedure that is very safe and entirely painless. Before having an MRI scan, all patients are asked to complete a form and it is necessary for the radiographer to be made aware of the presence of any metal, such as a pin in a limb, that may be present within the body. (This type of information will almost always be available from medical records.) All jewellery must be removed before having the scan and it is necessary to wear clothing that contains no metal (zips or buttons) or alternatively, a hospital gown. In some circumstances, the patient may be asked not to eat or drink anything in the hours before the scan. In others, a special contrast dye may be given by injection before the scan to more clearly highlight certain tissues and blood vessels.

Anyone who is to undergo MRI is encouraged beforehand to ask questions about the procedure and talk about any feelings of anxiety. If a person is very nervous and/or claustrophobic or if the patient is a young child who may not be able to remain still, it may be possible to have a sedative administered before having the scan.

Results are studied and interpreted by a specialist radiographer who then passes the results to the patient's consultant. They are usually available within about two weeks and the follow-up consultation normally takes place quite quickly, within a further 2 to 4 weeks. An MRI scan is a useful means of obtaining a direct picture of what is happening within a patient's back. It may point to the likely cause of pain but this is by no means certain in all cases.

Computerized axial tomography or computed tomography or CT scan

A CT scanning machine emits a series of narrow x-ray beams through the area of the body being scanned, tracing the shape of an arc. A succession of images ('slices') known as 'tomograms' are produced and these can be combined by a computer to produce a highly detailed, cross-sectional image. The CT scan is entirely painless and is useful for obtaining images of all the different types of internal organs and tissues. In the case of the spine, the scan can provide a highly detailed, three-dimensional view of vertebrae and intervertebral discs. It also provides an alternative means of scanning for patients who cannot undergo an MRI, eg those fitted with an internal heart pacemaker.

Before having a CT scan, it is necessary to remove jewellery and any clothing that might contain metal fastenings. Sometimes, a contrast dye is given, usually by means of injection, before having the scan and this is to show up certain tissues more clearly.

The CT scanner is a large machine with a central, circular hole. The patient lies, usually on his or her back, on a motorized bed and this is then moved forwards and backwards through the hole while the images are taken. The machine is operated remotely by a radiographer stationed in an adjacent room. The radiographer can see what is happening through a glass window and communication is maintained by means of an intercom system. The patient is asked to lie still while the machine is operating and the procedure usually lasts for anything up to 30 minutes.

A CT scan is by no means a routine procedure for people with back pain and is only likely to be carried out in a limited range of circumstances.

Bone scan or scintigram
A bone scan is a specialized type of radiological investigation using a radioactive tracer isotope that emits gamma radiation, to reveal the state of bones. It is used to screen the bones and skeleton for signs of various diseases and conditions, including fractures and cancer. The radioactive isotope is usually given by means of an injection into a vein in the patient's arm. There follows a wait of 2 to 4 hours to allow time for the isotope to settle in bone tissues. During this period, the person is asked to drink at least two pints of fluid and to empty the bladder before being scanned, as this helps to produce a clearer image. Before having the scan, which is achieved using

a 'gamma camera', the person is asked to remove all jewellery and clothing that may contain metal items. For the duration of the procedure, which lasts for about 20 minutes to an hour and is entirely painless, the person either sits in a chair or lies on a bed.

A bone scan is a useful means of viewing the whole skeleton and identifying 'hot spots' or problem areas that require further investigation. It is not a usual procedure for back pain sufferers and is carried out only in particular circumstances when certain conditions apply.

Nerve conduction tests

Nerve conduction tests are usually performed on patients showing signs of nerve root compression, when the cause appears to be unrelated to disc protrusion or bulging. The tests are carried out by a neurophysiologist and involve positioning very fine needles into certain muscles in order to detect types of electrical activity. The signals obtained can help to determine the nature of nerve damage, for example, if more than one nerve root is involved. Nerve conduction tests are not routinely performed but can be a useful diagnostic aid in a minority of cases where specific conditions apply.

Discography

Discography is the name given to a type of investigative procedure that uses injections (*discograms*) to try and identify the exact source of pain, usually in situations where an MRI scan has highlighted the presence of a number of degenerated intervertebral discs and it is difficult to pinpoint which one is involved. More than one injection may be made directly into a suspect disc and the information obtained is normally then used to decide upon a (surgical) solution to the problem. Antibiotics are often given on a preventative basis to lessen the possibility of infection. The procedure is usually carried out in the x-ray department of a hospital on an outpatient basis. The patient is usually sedated but does not require a general anaesthetic. Each needle is inserted with the aid of x-ray control and a contrast dye is passed into the centre of each disc under investigation. The patient is asked to report on the nature and level of pain and in some cases, local anaesthetic or a steroid solution may be administered to relieve pain. At the end of the procedure, the needles are withdrawn and a dressing is applied to each injection site. There may be a follow-up CT scan to see where the contrast dye has penetrated. Some discomfort may be experienced but complications are rare. Patients are advised to immediately report any fever, heat or severe pain that develops following the procedure that might indicate infection, nerve inflammation or other soft tissue damage so that appropriate treatment can be given.

14. Medical Treatments for Back Pain

Medication

'Over-the-counter' drugs
Always read the label before taking any 'over-the-counter' medication and if in doubt about the medicine, consult your doctor or a pharmacist.

Paracetamol: Paracetamol is an analgesic and antipyretic preparation (one that reduces pain and fever respectively) and a non-narcotic drug. It is effective in relieving many forms of mild to moderate pain and in 'taking the edge off' more severe pain. Taken at the recommended dose, it is considered to be a safe medicine and one that does not cause any problems for the gastrointestinal system. A typical tablet or caplet contains 500 mg of paracetamol along with some other inactive ingredients and the recommended dose for adults and children aged over 12 years is 1 to 2 tablets swallowed with water every 4 hours. Paracetamol is also available in soluble form for those who find it difficult to swallow tablets. No more than 8 tablets should be taken in any

24-hour period. The dose should be half this amount for children aged 6 to 12 years and preparations formulated especially for younger children are also available. An overdose of paracetamol is dangerous and can cause serious liver damage. Medical help needs to be obtained immediately in the event of overdose. No other preparations containing paracetamol should be taken along with paracetamol tablets and it should not be taken in combination with ibuprofen or aspirin, except under medical advice.

A doctor should be consulted before taking paracetamol if any of the following prescription drugs are being used: anticoagulants such as warfarin that 'thin' the blood; antiemetics (anti-sickness pills) such as domperidone and metclopramide; the antibiotic chloramphenicol; preparations to lower cholesterol such as cholestyramine. However, under medical advice, paracetamol is sometimes used as an 'in between' painkiller for patients taking other prescription medication. Paracetamol is also a component of many other prescribed, compound analgesic medications. Side effects are rare but you should stop taking paracetamol if you develop an unexpected allergic reaction such as a skin rash or experience any other unusual symptoms. In extremely rare cases, paracetamol can have effects upon the liver, kidneys or pancreas or cause blood changes but these are very unlikely to occur.

Ibuprofen: Ibuprofen belongs to the class of analgesic preparations known as non-steroidal anti-inflammatory drugs or NSAIDs. It is marketed under many different names and in different guises, including tablets, capsules, soluble, effervescent granules, syrup, slow-release tablets, and sprays, mousses and gels designed to be applied externally and rubbed onto the skin. Ibuprofen acts to reduce inflammation and counteract mild to moderate pain. It is widely used for back pain and arthritic and joint pains, headache, soft tissue injuries, period pain and postoperative pain. It is also used as a component of stronger, compound analgesic preparations containing opiates such as *codeine*. Dosages vary in strength and a single unit (tablet or capsule) may contain anything from 200 mg to 600 mg of ibuprofen. A typical adult dose is 1200 to 1800 mg each day in divided doses taken with food. Oral doses should not be taken if an externally applied cream or gel containing ibuprofen is being used at the same time. Ibuprofen has been known to react with certain other drugs, including quinolones, anticoagulants, such as warfarin, and thiazide diuretics. It should not be taken by people with a known allergy to aspirin or NSAIDs or by those with a peptic ulcer. It must be used cautiously by the elderly, pregnant and nursing women, those with gastrointestinal disorders, asthma, heart, liver or kidney disease, those with a history of heart failure or in persons with high blood pressure. Possible side effects include a skin rash, gastrointestinal upset and bleeding, and low levels of blood platelets affecting the blood's ability to form clots. Anyone experiencing unusual symptoms should stop taking ibuprofen and seek medical advice.

Aspirin: Aspirin or acetylsalicylic acid belongs to a group known as the salicylic drugs and is an analgesic, nonsteroidal anti-inflammatory and antipyretic preparation that, in its original form (derived from willow bark) has been used by mankind for many centuries. It is still widely used worldwide to relieve pain and fever but in Western countries, including the UK, it is given in low doses to thin the blood and reduce the risk of heart attack and stroke, more especially in the case of those who have already experienced a heart attack. It is generally available as capsules or tablets or as soluble tablets at a typical strength per tablet of 300 mg; tablets may be enteric-coated to protect the gut. The usual adult dose is 1 to 3 tablets every 4 hours with a maximum of 12 tablets in divided doses in any 24-hour period. It is usually recommended that tablets should be taken before meals or with food.

Aspirin is used for the relief of back pain, rheumatic, muscle and joint pain, headache, period pain and feverish illnesses such as colds and influenza. It should not be taken by children aged under 16 years, breastfeeding women, those who have an active peptic ulcer or who have experienced a peptic ulcer in the past, people with low prothrombin levels in the blood or haemophilia, those with known allergy to anti-inflammatory drugs or aspirin or with conditions of abnormal blood coagulation. Aspirin must be used with caution in patients with a history of bronchospasm or in those with high blood pressure. Aspirin may produce side effects that include gastrointestinal intolerance and bleeding and allergic and asthmatic responses. Anyone who experiences side effects should not take aspirin and should obtain medical advice. Aspirin may react with a number of other drugs: uricosuric agents, corticosteroids, coumarin anticoagulants, some other anti-inflammatories, hypoglycaemic drugs especially sulphonylureas, methotrexate, antacids, sodium valproate, sulfonamides, phenytoin and spironolactone.

Paracodol, Panadol Ultra and Solpadeine Max: These three preparations contain a combination of paracetamol and codeine phosphate (also known as *co-codamol*). Codeine phosphate belongs to the family of opiate-based or opiod drugs and it is a stronger analgesic than paracetamol and works in a different way, by mimicking the effects of pain-relieving endorphins that are naturally produced within the brain and spinal cord. Codeine phosphate combines with endorphin receptors in the central nervous system and acts to block transmission of pain signals. It is present in very small amounts in all three of these compound preparations, at 8 mg per tablet in Paracodol and 12.8 mg in Panadol Ultra and Solpadeine Max. All three contain the same amount of paracetamol per tablet, 500 mg.

These preparations, available as tablets or capsules, are effective in the relief of mild to moderate back pain, arthritic and rheumatic pain, strains and sprains and also headache, toothache, sinusitis, period pain and infections such as sore throat, fever, cold and influenza. The adult dose is 1 to 2 tablets every 4 hours, with no more than 8 tablets being taken in any 24-hour period. The tablets are not suitable for children aged under 12 years and should not be combined with any other preparations containing paracetamol. The same cautions apply as for paracetamol and pregnant or breastfeeding women should seek medical advice before taking these preparations. The tablets should not be used for more than 3 days without obtaining medical advice and patients with impaired liver or kidney function should ask a doctor before using them. Possible side effects include skin rash or allergic response, constipation, dizziness, drowsiness and nausea. If any of these are experienced, the tablets should be stopped immediately. Patients taking MAOIs (monoamine oxidase inhibitors), such as certain antidepressants, or cholesterol-lowering preparations, such as cholestyramine, or domperidone or metclopramide, or anticoagulants, such as warfarin, must use these preparations with care.

Prescription drugs

Codeine phosphate: Codeine phosphate is an opiate-based analgesic generally used in combination with paracetamol for the relief of back pain under the name of co-codamol. Co-codamol is for the most part a generic name (not a brand name) and it is available on prescription in various strengths to treat moderate back pain, with somewhat higher levels of codeine than those contained in the OTC preparations described above. It is available as tablets, capsules and effervescent tablets that can be dissolved in water and is also marketed as a brand named product called Codipar. (Stronger brand-name combinations are also available on prescription, used for severe pain but not commonly for back pain, including Kapake, Tylex and Solpadol.) Codeine may also be combined with ibuprofen to treat moderate back pain, such as in the preparation known as Codafen Continus. Prescription co-codamol tablets contain 500 mg of paracetamol and 15 mg to 20 mg of codeine phosphate. The adult dose is 1 to 2 tablets every 4 hours with a maximum dose of 8 tablets in any 24-hour period. The tablets are generally not suitable for children aged under 12 years and must not be used in patients with head injury or raised pressure within the skull, depressed respiration, obstructive airways disease, paralytic ileus (lack of movement of products of digestion through the gut) or acute alcoholism.

They must be taken with caution by pregnant and breastfeeding women or those in labour, elderly persons, debilitated persons, people with inflammation/obstruction of the bowel or inflammatory bowel disorders, men with enlarged prostate gland, those with an underactive thyroid gland, patients on sodium-restricted diets, those who have had recent bowel surgery, people with low blood pressure, lowered adrenal gland function (Addison's disease), epilepsy or urinary obstruction.

Possible drug interactions include MAOIs (monoamine oxidase inhibitors) and preparations that depress the central nervous system. Possible side effects include dizziness, drowsiness, dry mouth, constipation, breathlessness, skin rash, low heart beat rate, nausea, blurring of vision and contraction of pupils, retention of urine, confusion, tolerance and dependence, especially with prolonged use. If drowsiness occurs, do not drive or operate machinery. If constipation is experienced, the doctor may prescribe a laxative preparation (Movicol) and this is especially important for people with low back pain to avoid exacerbating the problem.

Diclofenac sodium: Diclofenac sodium is a non-steroidal, anti-inflammatory preparation (NSAID), phenylacetic acid, available in generic form and also in a number of brand-name preparations, including Arthrotec, Dicloflex, Diclomax, Moitifene, Solaraze, Volraman, Volsaid Retard, Voltarol, Voltarol Emulgel (available 'over-the-counter' as a rub-in gel, applied externally to the skin). Diclofenac sodium is available in various forms: tablets, capsules, sustained-release tablets, dispersible tablets for dissolving in water, suppositories and in ampoules for injection. Strengths vary from between 12.5 mg to 25 mg and 50 mg to 100 mg, depending upon the type of preparation and means of delivery. Tablets and capsules taken by mouth are usually enteric-coated. Typical oral dosages for adults are between 75 mg to 150 mg each day in 2 to 3 divided doses.

Diclofenac is used to relieve acute back pain, osteoarthritis, rheumatoid arthritis, ankylosing spondylitis, JRA, renal colic, fracture pain, acute gout, orthopaedic pain and traumatic back pain. Diclofenac is only used in special circumstances in children. It should not be used in people with a known allergy to NSAIDs or aspirin or those with a stomach ulcer. It must be used cautiously in elderly patients, pregnant or breastfeeding women, patients with impaired liver, kidney or heart function, porphyria (an inherited metabolic disorder), history of gastrointestinal lesions, blood abnormalities, asthma, high blood pressure or heart failure. Patients receiving long-term treatment must be monitored. Possible drug interactions may occur with lithium, anticoagulants, cardiac glycosides, diuretics, digoxin, methotrexate, salicylates, cyclosporin, oral hypoglycaemics (preparations to lower blood sugar levels), NSAIDs, steroids, mifepristone, quinolones and antihypertensives (drugs that lower blood pressure). Possible side effects include short-lived stomach pain, fluid retention, headache, gastrointestinal upset. In rare cases, there may be stomach ulcer, skin reactions, blood changes, disorders of the liver and kidney function.

Tramadol hydrochloride: An analgesic and opiate preparation available in generic form and also as branded products, including Tramake, Zamadol and Zydol. Drugs of the opiate family are derived from opium and include codeine and morphine. They act by depressing the central nervous thus relieving pain. Tramadol is available as tablets, sustained release capsules and sachets containing granules to be dissolved in water in various strengths from 50 mg to 200 mg. It can also be given as an intravenous injection and it is used to relieve moderate to severe (back) pain. The dosages depend upon individual circumstances and tramadol should be taken as directed by a doctor. A usual dose might be 50 mg to 100 mg, twice daily to start, increasing to 150 mg to 200 mg twice each day if needed to a maximum daily dose of 400 mg; 50 mg strength tablets may be taken every 4 to 6 hours to a total daily maximum of 8 tablets. Tramadol is not suitable for children or for pregnant or breastfeeding women. It must be used cautiously in elderly patients and in those who have previously suffered fits, depressed respiration, raised intracranial pressure (within the skull), seriously impaired liver or kidney function or people with previous history of drug dependency or abuse. Possible side effects include allergic reactions, itching, nettle rash, effects upon the central nervous system, gastrointestinal upset and profuse sweating, and, in rare cases, anaphylaxis, fainting, blood changes, severe rash, flushing, fits, depression of respiration, effects on heart and circulation, severe depression and feelings of anguish. Tramadol has been known to interact with SSRIs (selective serotonin re-uptake inhibitors), MAOIs (monoamine oxidase inhibitors), TCADs (tricyclic antidepressants), drugs that depress the central nervous system, carbamazepine and alcohol.

Diazepam: Diazepam is best known as a tranquillizer that is prescribed for the relief of extreme anxiety and as an anticonvulsant used to control severe epileptic fits. However, it can also have a useful role in reducing acute muscle spasm and it is for this function that it is sometimes prescribed for sort-term relief of severe back pain. Diazepam belongs to the family of drugs known as benzodiazepines and it acts upon GABA receptors in the central nervous system. GABA (gamma aminobutyric acid) is a naturally occurring neurotransmitter (a chemical that transmits electrical messages between nerve cells) and is the principle, fast-acting inhibitory neurotransmitter in the mammalian central brain and spinal cord. Diazepam stimulates the release of GABA, bringing about a calming and sedative response and in the case of muscles in spasm, causing suppression of excessive electrical activity and consequent relaxation. It is available in generic form and also under certain brand names, including Diazemuls, Diazepam Rectubes,

Stesolid, Valclair. It is available as tablets or a liquid to be taken by mouth and also as an emulsion for rectal application and as an injection. Oral preparations are normally used to treat muscle spasm in back pain and the lowest dose tablets available are 2 mg strength and these can be halved, if necessary.

The lowest possible effective dose is prescribed and use is normally limited to one week as diazepam is addictive and can produce withdrawal symptoms if stopped suddenly. Hence if the medication is used for longer than this, it must be gradually stopped using tapered, decreasing doses day by day to avoid the occurrence of unwanted symptoms. Diazepam can affect dexterity and judgement and must be used cautiously in children, pregnant women, elderly patients, those with chronic liver or kidney disease, respiratory disorders, acute, narrow-angle glaucoma, depression, certain inherited blood disorders (porphyria), mental illness and personality disorders. Use should be avoided in breastfeeding women, women in labour, acute lung insufficiency, depression of respiration, sleep apnoea (breathing stopping momentarily while asleep), severe liver insufficiency, myasthenia gravis, phobias or obsessions, chronic psychosis.

Possible side effects include drowsiness and light-headedness (continuing into the following day), confusion, ataxia (loss of coordination), weakness, dizziness, vertigo, low blood pressure, blood changes, disturbance of vision, gastrointestinal upset, skin rash, headache, amnesia. Also, urine retention and changes in libido. Possible drug interactions include alcohol, depressants of central nervous system, anticonvulsants, sleeping tablets, tricyclic antidepressants (amitryptyline), MAOIs (monoamine oxidase inhibitors), antipsychotics, opiods (codeine, morphine), barbiturates (phenobarbitol), certain antihistamines (chlorphenamine). Phenytoin and rifampicin may lessen the effect of diazepam while other drugs – isoniazid, ritonavir, cometidine, fluvoxamine, disulfram, omeprazole – may enhance potency. Hence anyone taking these drugs may require an adjusted dose of diazepam. Diazepam may decrease the potency of levodopa (used to treat Parkinson's disease) and may have an effect upon levels of phenytoin in the blood. Caffeine and theophylline may interfere with the sedative effect of diazepam. Anyone experiencing sedative effects should not attempt to drive or operate machinery and for safety reasons, it is sensible to limit activity while taking diazepam.

Amitryptyline hydrochloride: Amitryptyline is a generic medicine that is best known as a tricyclic antidepressant (TCAD) used for the treatment of depression, available as tablets of various strengths. But it has been discovered that in low doses, it is also highly effective in relieving nerve pain. It is now quite commonly prescribed for people suffering from severe back pain with nerve involvement, especially when other medication has proved to be inadequate, although it is not licensed for this particular function. Amitryptyline prolongs the availability of certain neurotransmitters (serotonin and noradrenaline) and also acts on cholinergic receptors. It promotes relaxation, enhances mood and may cause drowsiness. Feelings of depression generated by intense pain and an accompanying lack of sleep are symptoms commonly experienced by people suffering from nerve root pain. As well as acting on the pain itself, amitryptyline aids relaxation and sleep but it is necessary to take the medicine for 2 to 4 weeks for it to build up in the system and take effect. A doctor may recommend a one-month trial of amitryptyline for a patient, to assess if there is likely to be any benefit. If drowsiness is experienced while taking amitryptyline, you should not drive or operate machinery and if the medicine is taken for a long period, it must be gradually withdrawn to avoid the occurrence of unwanted withdrawal symptoms.

The medicine must be used with caution in children, elderly patients, pregnant and breastfeeding women, Parkinson's disease, adrenal gland tumour, glaucoma, retention of urine, kidney disease, lowered liver function, constipation, epilepsy, enlarged prostate gland (in men), heart disease, overactive thyroid gland, suicidal thoughts, psychoses and patients receiving electroconvulsive therapy. Use should be avoided in people with heart and circulatory disease and arrhythmia, recent heart attack, depressed bone marrow function, certain inherited blood disorders (porphyria), severe liver disorder and those who have been, or are taking, an MAOI (monoamine oxidase inhibitor). There are a number of possible side effects including drowsiness, dry mouth, gastrointestinal disturbance, constipation, disturbance of vision, hyponatramia (low blood sodium levels), postural hypotension (sudden drop in blood pressure when rising up, causing giddiness), confusion, heart beat disturbances, sweating, skin rash, muscle twitches, nausea, urine retention, mood swings, headache, altered sense of taste and fits. Other drugs, including 'over-the-counter' remedies and herbal preparations may react with amitryptyline, either by enhancing or decreasing its effect or the likely occurrence of certain side effects. Hence it is important for patients to discuss possible drug interactions with the doctor, before beginning a course of amitryptyline.

Gabapentin: Gabapentin is a GABA analogue, a substance that mimics the activity of the neurotransmitter, gamma aminobutyric acid, in the central nervous system. GABA stabilizes electrical activity in the central nervous system and has a calming effect and gabapentin is a synthetic substance that acts in a similar manner. It is available in generic form as tablets or capsules of varying strengths, from 100 mg to 800 mg of gabapentin and also as the brand-named product, Neurontin. It is used to treat neuropathic (nerve) pain and epilepsy and may occasionally be prescribed for patients with nerve root involvement in severe back pain. Dosages vary according to the condition being treated but an adult dose might be 300 mg to begin with, gradually increasing, if required to a maximum of 800 mg taken 3 times each day. Gabapentin must be stopped gradually with reducing doses over a one-week period to avoid the occurrence of unwanted withdrawal symptoms. This medication must be used cautiously in children and adolescents, elderly persons, pregnant and breastfeeding women, kidney disease, patients receiving dialysis treatment, patients subject to absence seizures and those with psychoses. Use should be avoided in children aged under 6 years and anyone with a known allergy to gabapentin or certain rare, inherited conditions of galactose intolerance. Side effects include fatigue, ataxia (lack of coordination), dizziness, drowsiness, fever, pharyngitis, urinary tract infections, headache, tremors, double vision, confusion, loss of ability to speak clearly, gastrointestinal disturbances, numbness/tingling/'pins-and-needles', joint pains, skin rash, purpura (skin blotches due to minute bleeds), oedema (swelling of ankles and feet or face), shortness of breath, rise in blood pressure, anxiety, irritability, insomnia, depression, insomnia. Antacid preparations should not be taken with gabapentin and the herbal remedy, St John's wort, should also be avoided.

Morphine sulphate: An analgesic, opiate, controlled drug available in generic form and also as brand-name products, including Cyclimorph, Morcap SR, MST Continus, MXL, Oramorph, Sevredol, Morphgesic Sr and Zomorph. It is available in different forms, including tablets, capsules, dissolvable tablets, sustained-release tablets or capsules, liquid or syrup, and injection, and these are of different strengths, ranging from 10 mg to 200 mg of morphine sulphate. All are used for the relief and control of severe pain. Morphine is not commonly prescribed for back pain and is only likely to be used if other medications and treatment methods have failed to provide adequate relief and the patient remains in severe pain, probably nerve root pain. The treatment period is likely to be limited to as short a time as possible. An anti-sickness preparation is often prescribed for use with morphine. Doses vary according to individual need and morphine should be taken as advised by a doctor. A typical adult, starting dose might be 10 mg every 4 hours for severe, acute pain. Special care is needed in the elderly, underactive thyroid gland, enlarged prostate gland in men, liver or kidney disorders, reduced gut movement, lowered adrenal gland function, reduced respiratory function, raised intracranial pressure (within the skull), acute alcoholism and 4 hours before and 4 hours following surgery. Morphine should not be taken by pregnant or breastfeeding women, or by patients with paralytic ileus (loss of movement in a part of the digestive tract), obstructive airways disease, acute liver disease, severely depressed respiration, head injury and high intracranial pressure. Side effects include gastrointestinal upset and sickness, sedation, drowsiness and tolerance and addiction. Possible drug interactions include cimetidine, depressants of the central nervous system and MAOIs (monoamine oxidase inhibitors).

Spinal injections

Epidural steroid injection
An epidural spinal injection in the lumbar spine, into the epidural space around the dura mater (membrane) is the most common type. A similar injection can also be given lower down, between the sacrum and the coccyx, then known as caudal, or higher up, in the thoracic or cervical spine. The injections are normally given without

the guidance of fluoroscopy (contrast dye injected with x-ray control) and comprise a combination of a corticosteroid preparation and local anaesthetic. The most common condition treated by this means is a prolapsed disc with some degree of nerve root irritation and inflammation. The corticosteroid reduces irritation and inflammation while the local anaesthetic helps to numb pain. Epidural injections can provide effective pain relief for a variable period of time but quite often, the procedure may need to be repeated. The injection is given by an appropriately trained physician, usually at an outpatient clinic with resuscitation facilities on hand. Complications are rare but there is a slight risk of infection, bleeding, allergic response or toxicity and so the patient is advised to report any untoward symptoms that might arise following the procedure in order that appropriate treatment can be given as soon as possible.

Facet joint injections and facet joint radio frequency lesioning (denervation)

When it is suspected that facet joints might be responsible for pain, targeted injections administered with x-ray control are sometimes used, both to confirm the diagnosis and as a means of providing temporary relief. A combination of local anaesthetic and corticosteroid is injected and this may provide relief for a variable period of weeks or months or in younger patients, give an opportunity for healing and recovery to occur. If relief is short-lived, a procedure known as radio frequency lesioning may provide a longer-lasting solution. A radio frequency generator is used and a current passed through an electrode heats tissue surrounding nerve endings to a temperature varying between 42°C and 80°C, interrupting the transmission of pain signals. This procedure is carried out by a trained physician in an x-ray department on an outpatient basis. The patient is sedated during the course of the procedure but does not require a general anaesthetic. One or more fine needles (cannulae) containing electrodes are accurately positioned with the guidance of x-ray control and then the current is switched on, usually for about one minute for each electrode. A nurse remains with the patient throughout the procedure. There may be some soreness and discomfort afterwards, lasting for about one week and it can take up to three weeks for full pain relief to be achieved. The majority of sufferers experience a considerable reduction in their pain (between 60% and 90% less than previously) and this may persist for a variable period of time, from several months to in excess of one year.

Nerve root blocks

Nerve root blocks are highly targeted as opposed to the more 'scatter gun' approach of epidural injections. Nerve-root blocking is concentrated upon an individual nerve(s), normally one that is being compressed and it is administered with the benefit of x-ray, fluoroscopic control, usually following an MRI scan. The procedure is carried out in a similar setting as that outlined above for facet joints but as with epidural injections, a combination of a small amount of corticosteroid and local anaesthetic is delivered directly to the nerve. Similar small risks apply to this procedure as for epidural injections but effective pain control is normally achieved for a time, although this does not rule out the possible need for future intervention.

Trigger point injections or TPI

Trigger point injections describe those made into tight knots or bands of tense and painful muscle. A TPI must only be administered by a trained specialist and it is given on an outpatient basis. In some cases, a nerve root block may be given first, depending upon individual circumstances. A needle is inserted into the muscle and a small quantity of local anaesthetic is injected, sometimes in combination with corticosteroid. The injection is usually effective in bringing about relaxation of the muscle and relief of pain, generally in combination with specific exercises and physiotherapy.

Fibroproliferative or Prolotherapy

Prolotherapy is a controversial form of treatment, involving injections targeted at ligaments, especially those in the lumbar and sacral areas of the spine when these are believed to be contributing to chronic low back pain. The procedure involves repeated injections of an irritant solution combined with local anaesthetic and this is designed to provoke the formation of fibrous, scar tissue to stabilize and strengthen the back and eventually lead to a reduction in pain. It is normally combined with exercises and possibly spinal manipulation and corticosteroid injections. This type of therapy has been used for about 50 years, especially in North America, but its use remains controversial in the UK.

Back surgery

In the vast majority of cases, back surgery is only performed when there is no other realistic option and standard treatments are inadequate. Most patients who eventually undergo surgery have a chronic back problem and are often constantly suffering moderate to severe pain with impaired mobility and reduced quality of life. However, even in these circumstances, surgery is not suitable for everyone. Surgery is only offered if an orthopaedic surgeon is able to clearly identify a problem that is amenable to such a procedure and if it is felt that the patient will experience direct benefit from having the operation. Surgical procedures fall into one of two groups: *stabilization* and *decompression*. Perhaps not surprisingly, stabilization covers a group of procedures carried out to restore or improve the strength, stability and configuration of a spine weakened by degeneration and/or injury or by a deformity that may either be congenital or have been caused by accidental trauma. Decompression procedures are performed to relieve pressure on nerves. The line between the two types is by no means clear cut but rather a gradation. In practice in the operating theatre, many patients will have a combination of procedures including elements of both types of spinal surgery.

The main conditions for which spinal surgery is performed are: prolapsed disc with nerve root compression; spinal stenosis; fractures, either related to aging and osteoporosis or caused by accidental injury; spondylolis-thesis; removal of tumours; degenerated discs (in some cases).

Discetomy

Discetomy means the surgical removal of an interverte-bral disc and it may be partial or total. It is performed to remove a bulging or prolapsed disc and to relieve nerve compression. It is often combined with disc replacement and/or with spinal fusion. Disc replacement involves the use of one of a number of different types of innovative prosthetic devices that aim to restore normal shape and natural movement to a considerable extent. The mini-mum recovery period following discetomy is 6 weeks al-though a longer time must be allowed for recovery to be complete.

Spinal fusion

Spinal fusion involves fusing together two or more verte-brae, often following discetomy, fracture, spondylolisthe-sis or to correct a deformity. It involves the use of metal rods, screws or 'cages' (prosthetic implants) and may re-quire an auto-bone graft from the patient's own tissue or utilize a bone substitute such as tri-calcium phosphate to aid stabilization and healing. The recovery period varies according to the nature of the problem, the age of the patient and various other factors that might influence the outcome. A minimum period of 6 weeks is needed for post-operative healing but full recovery may be quite prolonged, extending to anything up to one year and with physiotherapy quite often required.

A more recent innovation utilizes a flexible prosthetic implant attached to the outside of the vertebrae along with a pedicle screw system, to bring about stabilization while preserving structural integrity and mobility.

Laminectomy

Laminectomy is performed to relieve nerve compression and involves surgery to trim and remove a portion of the lamina of a vertebra in order to create more space. Nerve compression has usually been caused by a bulging or prolapsed disc or by spinal stenosis. The recovery period from this procedure varies but is typically between 2 months and 6 months.

Vertebroplasty and balloon kyphoplasty

Vertebroplasty is a fairly new stabilization procedure, involving the injection of a cement-like substance into one or more vertebral bodies in order to treat compression fractures caused by osteoporosis. The procedure is carried out under x-ray control with the cement placed along the fracture line. Balloon kyphoplasty is an alternative procedure utilizing a balloon that is inserted into the vertebral body and then filled with 'cement'. To date, neither of these procedures is widely used in the UK.

Removal of tumours

In the case of surgery to remove a spinal tumour, the aim is to remove the growth or as much of it as is possible, without causing harm or damage to vertebral structures. In many cases, this type of surgery relieves nerve compression caused by the presence of the tumour.

Recovery times are variable, depending upon the nature of the tumour, the overall health of the patient and whether any other treatment, such as radiotherapy or chemotherapy, is likely to be needed. However, most patients experience immediate relief from the painful symptoms of nerve compression and improved quality of life during the post-operative period.

15. Complementary Therapies

Most of the complementary therapies in this section (acupuncture, osteopathy, chiropractic, Alexander technique, acupressure, aromatherapy and massage, and hydrotherapy) are primarily concerned with the treatment of the body through massage and manipulation, both of which can ease the pain and discomfort of back pain, and, with the approval of the person treating the back pain, they can for the most part be used in conjunction with conventional medicine. For many patients complementary therapies can be a great help and provide much relief but you should avoid any therapist who offers guaranteed success. As with conventional medicine, treatments for back pain involving complementary therapies will work for some people but not for others.

Acupuncture

Introduction
Acupuncture is an ancient Chinese therapy that involves inserting needles into the skin at specific points of the body. The word 'acupuncture' originated from a Dutch

physician, William Ten Rhyne, who had been living in Japan during the latter part of the 17th century, and it was he who introduced the practice to Europe. The term means literally 'prick with a needle'. The earliest textbook on acupuncture, dating from approximately 400 BC, was called *Nei Ching Su Wen*, which means 'Yellow Emperor's Classic of Internal Medicine'. Also recorded at about the same time was the successful saving of a patient's life by acupuncture, the person having been expected to die whilst in a coma. Legend has it that acupuncture was developed when it was realized that soldiers who recovered from arrow wounds were sometimes also healed of other diseases from which they were suffering. Acupuncture was very popular with British doctors in the early 1800s for pain relief and to treat fever. Around the same time there was also a specific article that appeared in *The Lancet* on the successful treatment of rheumatism through acupuncture. Until the end of the Ching dynasty in China in 1911, acupuncture was slowly developed and improved, but then medicine from the West increased in popularity. However, more recently there has been a revival of interest and it is again widely practised throughout China. Also, nowadays the use of laser beams and electrical currents are found to give an increased stimulative effect when using acupuncture needles.

The specific points of the body into which acupuncture needles are inserted are located along 'meridians' (*see* Fig 11). These pathways or energy channels are believed to be related to the internal organs of the body. The energy is known as *qi* and the needles are used to decrease or increase its flow or to unblock it if it is impeded. Traditional Chinese medicine sees the body as being comprised of two natural forces known as *yin* and *yang*. These two forces are complementary to each other but also opposing. The yin is the female force and it is calm and passive representing the dark, cold, swelling and moisture. The yang is the male force and it is stimulating and aggressive, representing the heat and light, contraction and dryness. It is believed that the cause of ailments and diseases is due to an imbalance of these forces in the body, eg if a person is suffering from a headache or hypertension then this is because of an excess of yang. If, however, there is an excess of yin, this might result in tiredness, fluid retention and feeling cold.

The aim of acupuncture is to establish whether there is an imbalance of yin and yang and to rectify it by using the needles at certain points on the body. Traditionally there were 365 points but more have been found and nowadays there can be as many as 2,000. There are 14 meridians called after the organs they represent, eg the lung, kidney, heart and stomach as well as two organs unknown in orthodox medicine: the triple heater or warmer which relates to the activity of the endocrine glands and the control of temperature; and the pericardium which is concerned with seasonal activity and also regulates the circulation of the blood. Of the 14 meridians, there are two, known as the *du,* or governor, and the *ren*, or conception, which both run straight up the body's midline, although the du is much shorter, extending from the head down to the mouth, while the ren starts at the chin and extends to the base of the trunk.

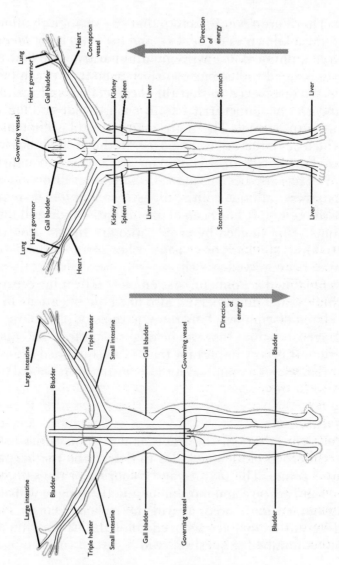

Fig 11 The main meridians of the body

There are several factors that can change the flow of qi (also known as *shi* or *ch'i*), and they can be of an emotional, physical or environmental nature. The flow may be changed to become too slow or fast, or it can be diverted or blocked so that the incorrect organ is involved and the acupuncturist has to ensure that the flow returns to normal. There are many painful afflictions for which acupuncture can be used. In the West, it has been used primarily for rheumatism, back pain and arthritis, but it has also been used to alleviate other disorders such as stress, allergy, colitis, digestive troubles, insomnia, asthma, etc. It has been claimed that withdrawal symptoms (experienced by people who are in the process of stopping smoking or ceasing other forms of addiction) have been helped as well.

Qualified acupuncturists complete a training course of three years' duration and also need qualifications in the related disciplines of anatomy, pathology, physiology and diagnosis before they can belong to a professional association. It is very important that a fully qualified acupuncturist, who is a member of the relevant professional body, is consulted.

Treatment

At a consultation, the traditional acupuncturist uses a set method of ancient rules to determine the acupuncture points. The texture and colouring of the skin, type of skin, posture and movement and the tongue will all be examined and noted, as will the patient's voice. These different factors are all needed for the Chinese diagnosis. A number of questions will be asked concerning the diet, amount of exercise taken, lifestyle, fears and phobias, sleeping patterns and reactions to stress. Each wrist has six pulses, and each of these stand for a main organ and its function. The pulses are felt (known as palpating), and by this means acupuncturists are able to diagnose any problems relating to the flow of qi and if there is any disease present in the internal organs. The first consultation may last an hour, especially if detailed questioning is necessary along with the palpation.

The needles used in acupuncture are disposable and made of a fine stainless steel and they come already sealed in a sterile pack. They can be sterilized by the acupuncturist in a machine known as an autoclave but using boiling water is not adequate for this purpose. (Diseases such as HIV and hepatitis can be passed on by using unsterilized needles.) Once the needle is inserted into the skin it is twisted between the acupuncturist's thumb and forefinger to spread or draw the energy from a point. The depth to which the needle is inserted can vary from just below the skin to up to 12 mm (half an inch) and different sensations may be felt, such as a tingling around the area of insertion or a loss of sensation at that point. Up to 15 needles can be used but around 5 are generally sufficient. The length of time that they are left in varies from a few minutes to half an hour and this is dependent on a number of factors such as how the patient has reacted to previous treatment and the ailment from which he or she is suffering.

Patients can generally expect to feel an improvement after 4 to 6 sessions of therapy, the beneficial effects occurring gradually, particularly if the ailment has obvious and long-standing symptoms. Other diseases, such as asthma, will probably take longer before any definite improvement is felt. It is possible that some patients may not feel any improvement at all, or even feel worse after the first session and this is probably due to the energies in the body being over-stimulated. To correct this, the acupuncturist will gradually use fewer needles and for a shorter period of time. If no improvement is felt after about 6 to 8 treatments, then it is doubtful whether acupuncture will be of any help. For general body maintenance and health, most traditional acupuncturists suggest that sessions be arranged at the time of seasonal changes.

How does it work?

There has been a great deal of research, particularly by the Chinese, who have produced many books detailing a high success rate for acupuncture in treating a variety of disorders. These results are, however, viewed cautiously in the West as methods of conducting clinical trials vary from East to West. Nevertheless trials have been carried out in the West and it has been discovered that a pain message can be stopped from reaching the brain using acupuncture. The signal would normally travel along a nerve but it is possible to 'close a gate' on the nerve, thereby preventing the message from reaching the brain, hence preventing the perception of pain. Acupuncture is believed to work by blocking the pain signal. However, doctors stress that pain can be a warning that something is wrong or of the occurrence of a particular disease, such as cancer, that requires an orthodox remedy or method of treatment.

It has also been discovered that there are substances produced by the body that are connected with pain relief. These substances are called endorphins and encephalins, and they are natural opiates. Studies from all over the world show that acupuncture stimulates the release of these opiates into the central nervous system, thereby giving pain relief. The amount of opiates released has a direct bearing on the degree of pain relief. Acupuncture is a widely used form of anaesthesia in China where, for suitable patients, it is said to be extremely effective (90 %). It is used successfully during childbirth, dentistry and for operations. Orthodox doctors in the West now accept that heat treatment, massage and needles used on a sensitive part of the skin afford relief from pain caused by disease elsewhere. These areas are known as trigger points, and they are not always situated close to the organ that is affected by disease. It has been found that approximately three quarters of these trigger points are the same as the points used in Chinese acupuncture. Recent research has also shown that it is possible to find the acupuncture points with electronic instruments as they register less electrical resistance than other areas of skin. As yet, no evidence has been found to substantiate the existence of meridians.

Osteopathy

Introduction

Osteopathy is an alternative medical treatment that uses manipulation and massage to help distressed muscles and joints and make them work smoothly. The profession began in 1892 when Dr Andrew Taylor Still (1828–1917), an American farmer, inventor and doctor, opened the USA's first school of osteopathic medicine. He sought alternatives to the medical treatments of his day which he believed were ineffective as well as often harmful.

Still's new philosophy of medicine, based upon the teachings of Hippocrates, advocated that 'Finding health should be the purpose of a doctor. Anyone can find disease.' Like Hippocrates, Still recognized that the human body is a unit in which structure, function, mind and spirit all work together. The therapy aims to pinpoint and treat any problems that are of a mechanical nature. The body's frame consists of the skeleton, muscles, joints and ligaments and all movements or activities such as running, swimming, eating, speaking and walking depend upon it.

Still came to believe that it would be safer to encourage the body to heal itself, rather than use the drugs that were then available and that were not always safe. He regarded the body from an engineer's point of view and the combination of this and his medical experience of anatomy, led him to believe that ailments and disorders could occur when the bones or joints no longer functioned in harmony. He believed that manipulation was the cure for the problem. Although his ideas provoked at first a great deal of opposition from the American medical profession, they slowly came to be accepted. The bulk of scientific research has been done in America with a number of medical schools of osteopathy being established. Dr Martin Littlejohn, who was a pupil of Dr Still, brought the practice of osteopathy to the UK around 1900, with the first school being founded in 1917 in London. He emphasized the compassionate care and treatment of the person as a whole, not as a collection of symptoms or unrelated parts. The philosophy and practices of A. T. Still, considered radical in the 1800s, are generally accepted principles of good medicine today.

Treatment

In osteopathy, it is believed that if the basic framework of the body is undamaged, then all physical activities can be accomplished efficiently and without causing any problems. The majority of an osteopath's patients suffer from disorders of the spine, which result in pain in the lower part of the back and in the neck. As has already been established, a great deal of pressure is exerted on the spinal column, and especially on the cartilage between the individual vertebrae. This is a constant pressure due to the effects of gravity that occurs merely by standing. If a person stands incorrectly with stooped shoulders, this could exacerbate any existing problems or perhaps initiate new ones.

Problems that prevent the body from working correctly or create pain can be due to injury or stress. Injuries to muscles or joints, such as the ankle, hip, wrist or elbow, can benefit from treatment by osteopathy and where there is lower back pain and neck pain osteopathy can often ease matters considerably. During treatment, the joints and framework of the body are manipulated and massaged where necessary so that the usual action is regained. Stress can result, for example, in what is known as a 'tension headache' since the stress experienced causes a contraction of the muscles at the back of the neck.

Again relief can be obtained through manipulation and massage.

To find a fully qualified osteopath, it is advisable to contact the relevant professional body, or your GP may be able to help. At the first visit to an osteopath, he or she will need to know the complete history of any problems experienced, how they first occurred and what eases or aggravates matters. A patient's case history and any form of therapy that is currently in use will all be of relevance to the practitioner. A thorough examination will then take place observing how the patient sits, stands or lies down and also the manner in which the body is bent to the side, back or front. As each movement takes place, the osteopath is able to take note of the extent and ability of the joint to function. The practitioner will also feel the muscles, soft tissues and ligaments to detect if there is any tension present. Whilst examining the body, the osteopath will note any problems that are present and, as an aid to diagnosis, use may also be made of checking reflexes, such as the knee-jerk reflex. If a patient has been involved in an accident, x-rays can be checked to determine the extent of any problem. It is possible that a disorder will not benefit from treatment by osteopathy and the patient would be advised accordingly. If this is not the case, treatment can commence with the chosen course of therapy.

There is no set number of consultations necessary, as this will depend upon the nature of the problem and also for how long it has been apparent. It is possible that a severe disorder that has arisen suddenly can be alleviated at once. The osteopath is likely to recommend a number of things so that patients can help themselves between treatments. For example, techniques such as learning to relax, how to stand and sit correctly and additional exercises might be suggested by the osteopath. Patients generally find that each consultation is quite pleasant and they feel much more relaxed and calm afterwards. The length of each session can vary, but it is generally in the region of half an hour.

How does it work?
As the osteopath gently manipulates the joint, it will lessen any tenseness present in the muscles and also improve its ability to work correctly and to its maximum extent. It is this manipulation that can cause a clicking noise to be heard. As well as manipulation, other methods such as massage can be used to good effect. Muscles can be freed from tension if the tissue is massaged and this will also stimulate the flow of blood. In some cases, the patient may experience a temporary deterioration once treatment has commenced, and this is more likely to occur if the ailment has existed for quite some time.

People who have to spend a lot of their life driving are susceptible to a number of problems related to the manner in which they are seated. If their position is incorrect they can suffer from tension headaches, pain in the back and the shoulders and neck can feel stiff. There are a number of ways in which these problems can be remedied such as holding the wheel in the approved manner (at roughly 'ten to two' on the dial of a clock). The arms should not be held out straight and stiff, but should feel relaxed and with the arms bent at the elbow. In order that the driver can maintain a position in which the back and neck feel comfortable, the seat should be moved so that it is tilting backwards a little, although it should not be so far away that the pedals are not easily reached. The legs should not be held straight out, and if the pedals are the correct distance away the knees should be bent a little and feel quite comfortable. It is also important to sit erect and not slump in the seat. The driver's rear should be positioned right at the back of the seat and this should be checked each time before using the vehicle. It is also important that there is adequate vision from the mirror so its position should be altered if necessary.

If the driver already has a back problem then it is a simple matter to provide support for the lower part of the back. If this is done it should prevent strain on the shoulders and backbone. Whilst driving, the person should make a conscious effort to ensure that the shoulders are not tensed, but held in a relaxed way. Another point to remember is that the chin should not be stuck out but kept in, otherwise the neck muscles will become tensed and painful. Drivers can perform some beneficial exercises while they are waiting in a queue of traffic. To stretch the neck muscles, put the chin right down on to the chest and then relax. This stretching exercise should be done several times. While driving, simply contracting and relaxing the muscles in the stomach will have a positive effect on the flow of blood to the legs and also will improve how a person is seated. Another exercise involves raising the shoulders upwards and then moving them backwards in a circular motion. The head should also be inclined forward a little. This should also be done several times to gain the maximum effect.

Fig 12 below illustrates an example of treatment by manipulation, in which the osteopath works on a knee that has been injured. To first determine the extent of the problem, the examination will be detailed and any previous accidents or any other relevant details will be requested. If the practitioner concludes that osteopathy will be of benefit to the patient, the joint will be manipulated so that it is able to function correctly and the manipulation will also have the effect of relaxing the muscles that have become tensed due to the injury.

Another form of therapy, which is known as cranial osteopathy, can be used for patients suffering from pain

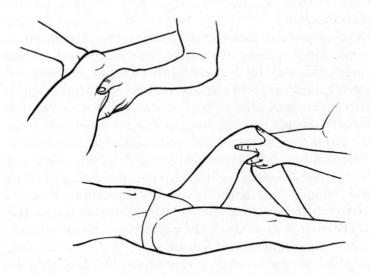

Fig 12 Osteopathic treatment of the knee using manipulation

in the face or head. This is effected by the osteopath using slight pressure on these areas including the upper part of the neck. If there is any tautness or tenseness present, the position is maintained while the problem improves. It is now common practice for doctors to recommend some patients to use osteopathy and some GPs use the therapy themselves after receiving training. Although its benefits are generally accepted for problems of a mechanical nature, doctors believe it is vital that they first decide upon what is wrong before any possible use can be made of osteopathy.

Chiropractic

Introduction

The word chiropractic originates from two Greek words: *kheir* which means 'hand' and *praktikos* which means 'practical'. A school of chiropractic was established in about 1895 by a healer called Daniel Palmer (1845–1913). He was able to cure a man's deafness that had occurred when he bent down and felt a bone click. Upon examination, Palmer discovered that some bones in the man's spine had become displaced. After successful manipulation the man regained his hearing. Palmer formed the opinion that if there was any displacement in the skeleton this could affect the function of nerves, either increasing or decreasing their action and thereby resulting in a malfunction, ie a disease.

Chiropractic is used to relieve pain by manipulation and to correct any problems that are present in joints and muscles but especially the spine. As in osteopathy, no

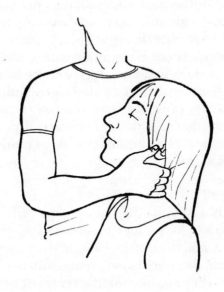

Fig 13 Chiropractic manipulation of the neck

use is made of surgery or drugs. The majority of a chiropractor's patients suffer from neck and back pain. For example, people suffering from whiplash injuries sustained in car accidents commonly seek the help of a chiropractor. Another common problem that chiropractors treat is headaches, and it is often the case that tension caused by stress is the underlying cause as it makes the neck muscles contract.

Athletes can also obtain relief from injuries such as tennis elbow, pulled muscles, injured ligaments and sprains, etc at the hands of a chiropractor. As well as the

181

normal methods of manipulating joints, the chiropractor may decide it is necessary to use applications of ice
or heat to relieve the injury.

Although there is quite a small number of chiropractors in the UK, there is a degree of contact and liaison between them and doctors. It is generally accepted that
chiropractic is an effective remedy for spinal and muscular problems, and the majority of doctors would be
happy to accept a chiropractor's diagnosis and treatment
in these areas.

Treatment

At the initial visit, the chiropractor will ask the patient
for details of his or her case history, including the present
problem, and during the examination painful and tender
areas will be noted and joints will be checked to see
whether they are functioning correctly or not. X-rays are
frequently used by chiropractors since they can show
signs of bone disease, fractures or arthritis as well as the
spine's condition. After the initial visit, any treatment
will normally begin as soon as the patient has been in-
formed of the chiropractor's diagnosis. If it has been decided that chiropractic therapy will not be of any benefit,
the patient will be advised accordingly.

For treatment, underwear and/or a robe will be worn,
and the patient will either lie, sit or stand on a specially
designed couch. Chiropractors use their hands in a skilful
way to effect the different manipulative techniques. If it is
decided that manipulation is necessary to treat a painful
lumbar joint, the patient will need to lie on his or her side.
The upper and lower spine will then be rotated manually

but in opposite ways. This manipulation will have the effect of partially locking the joint that is being treated, and the upper leg is usually flexed to aid the procedure. The vertebra that is immediately below or above the joint will then be felt by the chiropractor, and the combination of how the patient is lying, coupled with gentle pressure applied by the chiropractor's hand, will move the joint to its furthest extent of normal movement. There will then be a very quick push applied on the vertebra, which results in its movement being extended further than normal, ensuring that full use of the joint is regained. This is due to the muscles that surround the joint being suddenly stretched, which has the effect of relaxing the muscles of the spine that work upon the joint. This alteration should cause the joint to be able to be used more naturally and should not be a painful procedure.

There can be a variety of effects felt after treatment – some patients may feel sore or stiff, or may ache for some time after the treatment, while others will experience the lifting of pain at once. In some cases there may be a need for multiple treatments, perhaps four or more, before improvement is felt. On the whole, problems that have been troubling a patient for a considerable time (chronic) will need more therapy than anything that occurs quickly and is very painful (acute).

Children can also benefit from treatment by a chiropractor, as there may be some slight accident that has occurred in their early years that can reappear in adult life in the form of back pain. It can easily happen, for example, when a child learns to walk and bumps into furniture, or when a baby falls out of a cot. This could result in some damage to the spine that will only show up in adult life when they experience back pain. At birth, a baby's neck may be injured or the spine may be strained if the use of forceps is necessary, and this can result in headaches and neck problems as he or she grows to maturity. If a parent has any worries it is best to consult a doctor and it is possible that the child will be recommended to see a qualified chiropractor. To avoid any problems in adult life, chiropractors recommend that children have occasional examinations to detect any damage or displacement in bones and muscles.

As well as babies and children, adults of all ages can benefit from chiropractic. For example, there are some people who regularly take painkillers for painful joints or back pain, but this does not deal with the root cause of the pain, only the symptoms that are produced. Chiropractic could be of considerable help in giving treatment to these people. Many pregnant women experience backache at some stage during their pregnancy because of the extra weight that is placed on the spine. At the time of giving birth, changes take place in the pelvis and joints at the bottom of the spine and this can be a cause of back pain. Lifting and carrying babies, if not done correctly, can also damage the spine and thereby make the back painful.

It is essential that any chiropractor is fully qualified and registered with the relevant professional association.

The Alexander technique

Introduction
The Alexander technique is a practical and simple method of learning to focus attention on how we use

ourselves during daily activities. Frederick Mathias Alexander (1869–1955), an Australian therapist, demonstrated that the difficulties many people experience in learning, in control of performance, and in physical functioning are caused by unconscious habits. These habits interfere with our natural poise and capacity to learn. When we stop interfering with the innate coordination of the body, we can take on more complex activities with greater self-confidence and presence of mind. It is about learning to bring into our conscious awareness the choices we make, as we make them. Gentle hands-on and verbal instruction reveal the underlying principles of human coordination, allow the student to experience and observe their own habitual patterns, and give the means for release and change.

Most of us are unconsciously 'armouring' ourselves in relation to our environment. This is hard work and often leaves us feeling anxious, alienated, depressed and unlovable. Armouring is a deeply unconscious behaviour that has probably gone on since early childhood, maybe even since infancy. Yet it is a habit we can unlearn in the present through careful self-observation. We can unlearn our use of excess tension in our thoughts, movements, and relationships.

The Alexander technique is based on correct posture which allows the body to function naturally and with the minimum amount of muscular effort. F. M. Alexander was also an actor. He found that he was losing his voice when performing but after resting his condition temporarily improved. Although he received medical help, the condition was not cured and it occurred to him that while acting he might be doing something that caused the problem. To see what this might be he performed his act in front of a mirror and saw what happened when he was about to speak: he experienced difficulty in breathing and lowered his head, thus making himself shorter. He realized that the strain of remembering his lines and having to project his voice, so that the people furthest away in the audience would be able to hear, was causing him a great deal of stress and the way he reacted was a quite natural reflex action. In fact, even thinking about having to project his voice made the symptoms recur and from this he concluded that there must be a close connection between body and mind. He was determined to try and improve the situation and gradually, by watching and altering his stance and posture and his mental attitude to his performance on stage, matters improved. He was then able to act and speak on stage and use his body in a more relaxed and natural fashion. There has been scientific research carried out that concurs with the beliefs that Alexander formed, including the relationship between mind and body (eg the thought of doing an action actually triggering a physical reaction or tension).

In 1904 Alexander travelled to London where he decided to let others know about his method of retraining the body. He soon became very popular with other actors who appreciated the benefits of using his technique. Other public figures, including the author Aldous Huxley, also benefited. Later he went to America, achieving considerable success and international recognition for his technique. At the age of 78 he suffered a stroke but by using his method he managed to regain the use of all his faculties – an achievement that amazed his doctors.

Treatment
The Alexander technique is said to be completely harmless, encouraging an agreeable state between mind and body. It is also helpful for a number of disorders such as posture-related headaches and back pain. Learning the Alexander Technique can help to prevent or alleviate conditions associated with undue tension or poor posture. Examining the way people carry themselves and hold tension, and teaching them to move more naturally and freely, can address the underlying cause of many such problems. Today, Alexander training centres can be found all over the world and you can learn the Alexander Technique through one-to-one lessons with a qualified teacher who will address your individual needs. Learning the Alexander Technique involves changing long-standing habits of movement, and relies on your active participation, but achieving the correct posture and balance for the body so that it is well aligned needs very little muscular effort.

A simple test to determine if people can benefit from using the Alexander technique is to observe their posture (*see* Fig 14 on page 188). We frequently do not stand correctly and this can encourage aches and pains if the body is unbalanced. It is incorrect, for example, to stand with round shoulders or to slouch – this often looks and feels uncomfortable – but on the other hand we sometimes hold ourselves too erect and unbending, which can also have a bad effect on our health and well-being.

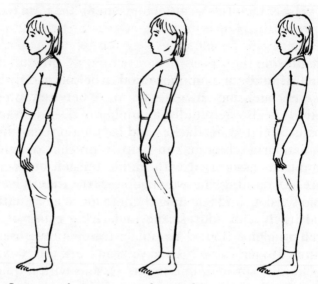

Fig 14a Incorrect and correct posture when standing

Many muscles are used in everyday activities, and over the years bad habits can develop unconsciously, with stress also affecting the use of muscles. This can be seen, for example, in people gripping a pen with too much force or holding the steering wheel of a car too tightly while driving. Muscular tension can be a serious problem affecting some people when the head, neck and back can be forced out of line, which in turn leads to rounded shoulders with the head held forward and the back curved. If this situation is not altered and the body is not correctly re-aligned, the spine may become curved leading to back pain and a strain on internal organs such as the chest and lungs.

Once a teacher has been consulted, all movements and how the body is used will be observed. An Alexander teacher helps people to use less tension as they move by monitoring their posture and reminding them to implement tiny changes in movement to eradicate the habit of excess tension. Patients learn to stop bracing themselves up or collapsing into themselves. As awareness grows, it becomes easier to recognize and relinquish the habit of armouring and dissolve the artificial barriers we put between ourselves and others.

The length of time for each lesson can vary from about 30 minutes to 45 minutes and the number of lessons is usually between 10 and 30, by which time people should have gained sufficient knowledge to continue practising the technique by themselves.

How does it work?

No force is used by the teacher other than some gentle manipulation to start people off correctly. Some teachers use light pushing methods on the back and hips, etc, while others might first ensure that you are relaxed and then pull gently on the neck, which stretches the body. Any bad postures will be corrected by the teacher and you will be shown how best to alter this so that you use your muscles more effectively and with the least effort. Any manipulation that is used will be to ease the body into a more relaxed and natural position. With frequent treatments for posture and the release of tension, your muscles and body should be functioning correctly, with a consequent improvement in, for example, how you are walking and sitting.

When it comes to walking, you should not slouch, hold your head down or have your shoulders stooped. The head should be balanced correctly above the spine with the shoulders relaxed. You should try to feel the weight of the body being transferred from one foot to the other while you are walking.

Where sitting is concerned, the Alexander technique can be applied to two positions adopted every day, namely sitting on a chair and sitting at a desk or table.

To be seated on a chair in the correct manner (*see* the figure on the right of Fig 14b below) your head should be comfortably balanced, with no tension in the shoulders. There should be a small gap between the knees and the soles of the feet should be flat on the floor (if your legs are crossed the spine and pelvis become out of line or twisted).

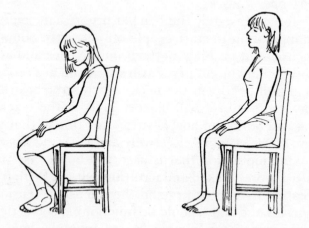

Fig 14b Incorrect and correct posture when sitting on a chair

It is incorrect to sit with your head lowered and the shoulders slumped forward because the stomach becomes restricted and your breathing may also be affected. On the other hand, it is also incorrect to hold your body in too stiff and erect a position.

To sit correctly while working at a table or a desk, your body should be held upright but in a relaxed manner with any bending movement coming from the hips and with your seat flat on the chair (*see* the figure on the right of Fig 14c below). A pen should be held lightly if writing and if using a computer you should ensure that your arms are relaxed and feel comfortable. The chair should be set at a comfortable height with regard to the level of the desk. You should try not to hold your arms in a tense, tight manner nor should you lean forward over a desk because this can hamper your breathing.

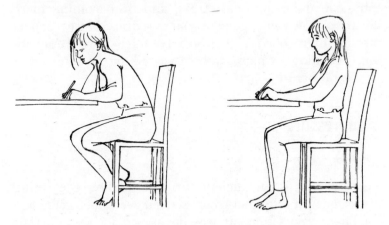

Fig 14c Incorrect and correct posture when sitting at a desk

Once someone has learned how to improve their posture, they carry their body in a more upright way and appear taller. The technique has been found to be of benefit to dancers, athletes and people who have to speak in public. Other disorders claimed to have been treated successfully are depressive states, back pain and headaches caused by tension, anxiety, hypertension, respiratory problems, colitis, osteoarthritis and rheumatoid arthritis, and sciatica. The Alexander technique is recommended for people of all ages, as learning how to resist stress can improve our overall quality of life, both mental and physical.

Although the Alexander technique does not treat specific symptoms, you can encourage a marked improvement in your overall health, alertness, and performance by consciously eliminating harmful habits that cause physical and emotional stress, and by becoming more aware of how you engage in your activities. Most teachers are members of STAT, the Society of Teachers of Alexander Technique, which can be accessed on the Internet at www.stat.org.uk.

Acupressure

Introduction

Acupressure is an ancient form of healing combining massage and acupuncture, practised over 3,000 years ago in Japan and China. It was developed into its current form using a system of special massage points and is today still practised widely in the Japanese home environment.

Certain 'pressure points' are located in various parts of the body and these are used by the practitioner by massaging firmly with the thumb or fingertip. These points are the same as those utilized in acupuncture. There are various ways of working and the pressure can be applied by the practitioner's fingers, thumbs, knees, palms of the hand, etc. Relief from pain can be quite rapid at times, depending upon its cause, while other more persistent problems can take longer to improve.

Acupressure is said to enhance the body's own method of healing, thereby preventing illness and improving the energy level. The pressure exerted is believed to regulate the energy or *qi* that flows along the body's meridians. As previously mentioned, the meridians are the invisible channels that run along the length of the body (*see* page 169). Specifically named meridian lines may also be used to treat ailments other than those relating to it.

Ailments claimed to have been treated successfully are back pain, asthma, digestive problems, insomnia, migraine and circulatory problems, amongst others. Changes in diet, regular exercise and certain self-checking methods may be recommended by your practitioner. It must be borne in mind that some painful symptoms are the onset of serious illness so you should always first consult your GP.

Treatment
Before any treatment commences, a patient will be

asked for details of their lifestyle and diet and the pulse rate will be taken along with any relevant past history relating to the current problem. The patient will be asked to lie on a mattress on the floor or on a firm table, and comfortable but loose-fitting clothing is best so that the practitioner can work most effectively on the energy channels. No oils are used on the body and there is no equipment. Each session lasts from approximately 30 minutes to an hour.

Once the pressure is applied, and this can be done in a variety of ways particular to each practitioner, varying sensations may be felt. Some points may feel sore or tender and there may be some discomfort such as a deep pain or coolness. However, it is believed that this form of massage works quickly so that any tenderness soon passes.

The number of treatments will vary from patient to patient, according to how they respond and what problem or ailment is being treated. Weekly visits may be needed if a specific disorder is being treated while other people may go whenever they feel in need. It is advisable for women who are pregnant to check with their practitioner first since some of the acupressure methods are not recommended during pregnancy.

Acupressure can be practised safely at home although it is usually better for one person to perform the massage on another. Common problems, such as headache, constipation and toothache, can be treated quite simply although there is the possibility, if the pressure points are overstimulated, of a problem worsening first before an improvement occurs. You should, however, see your doctor if any ailment persists. To treat headache, facial soreness, toothache and menstrual pain, locate the fleshy piece of skin between the thumb and forefinger and squeeze firmly, pressing towards the forefinger. The pressure should be applied for about 5 minutes and either hand can be used. This point is known as 'large intestine 4'.

To aid digestive problems in both adults and babies, eg to settle infantile colic, the point known as 'stomach 36' is utilized, which is located on the outer side of the leg about 75 mm (3 ins) down from the knee. This point should be quite simple to find as it can often feel slightly tender. It should be pressed quite firmly and strongly for about 5 to 10 minutes with the thumb.

How does it work?
Before treatment begins, the practitioner should ensure that the patient is warm, relaxed, comfortable and wearing loose-fitting clothing and that he or she is sitting in a special chair or lying on a firm mattress or couch. To discover the areas that need to be worked on, the practitioner will press firmly over the body and see which areas are tender. These tender areas on the body correspond to an organ that is not working correctly. To commence, they will massage the area that needs to be worked on using fingertips or thumbs – a pressure of about 4.5 kg (10 lbs) being exerted. The massage movements will be performed very quickly, about 50 to 100 times every minute, and some discomfort is likely (which will soon

pass) but there should be no pain. Particular care will be taken by the practitioner to avoid causing pain on the face, stomach or over any joints. If a baby or young child is being massaged then considerably less pressure will be used. Approximately 5 to 15 minutes is needed at each point for adults (but only about 30 seconds for babies or young children).

Using 'self-help' acupressure, massage can be repeated as often as is felt to be necessary with several sessions per hour usually being sufficient for painful conditions that have arisen suddenly. It is possible that as many as 20 sessions may be necessary for persistent conditions causing pain, with greater intervals of time between treatments as matters improve.

It is not advisable to try anything that is at all complicated and a trained practitioner will obviously be able to provide the best level of treatment and help. To contact a reputable practitioner who has completed the relevant training it is advisable to contact the appropriate professional body.

Aromatherapy

Introduction

Aromatherapy is a method of healing using very concentrated essential oils that are often highly aromatic and are extracted from plants. Constituents of the oils confer the characteristic perfume or odour given off by a particular plant. Essential oils help the plant in some way to complete its cycle of growth and reproduction. For example, some oils may attract insects for the purpose of pollination; others may render it distasteful as a source of food. Any part of a plant – the stems, leaves, flowers, fruits, seeds, roots or bark – may produce essential oils or essences but often only in minute amounts. Different parts of the same plant may produce their own form of oil. An example of this is the orange, which produces oils with different properties in the flowers, fruits and leaves.

Throughout the course of human history the healing properties of plants and their essential oils has been recognized and most people probably had some knowledge about their use. It was only with the great developments in science and orthodox medicine, particularly the manufacture of antibiotics and synthetic drugs, that knowledge and interest in the older methods of healing declined. However, more recently there has been a rekindling of interest in the practice of aromatherapy with many people turning to this form of treatment.

A wide range of conditions and disorders may benefit from aromatherapy and it is considered to be a gentle treatment suitable for all age groups. It is especially beneficial for long-term chronic conditions, such as back pain, and is of great benefit in relieving stress and stress-related symptoms such as anxiety, insomnia and depression.

Many of the essential oils can be safely used at home and the basic techniques of use can soon be mastered. However, some should only be used by a trained aromatherapist and others must be avoided in certain conditions such as pregnancy. In some circumstances, massage is not considered to be advisable and it is wise to seek medical advice in the event of doubt or if the ailment is more than a minor one.

Treatment

Aromatherapy is a holistic approach to healing hence the practitioner endeavours to build up a complete picture of the patient and his or her lifestyle, temperament and family circumstances, as well as noting the symptoms which need to be to be treated. Depending upon the picture that is obtained, the aromatherapist decides upon the essential oil or oils that are most suitable and likely to prove most helpful in the circumstances that prevail.

Aromatherapists can draw on their wide-ranging knowledge and experience to offer different methods of treatment using essential oils. Their most common treatment is massage but there are other treatments that we can use at home.

Massage

Massage is the most familiar method of treatment associated with aromatherapy. Essential oils are able to penetrate the skin and are taken into the body, exerting healing and beneficial influences on internal tissues and organs. The oils used for massage are first diluted by being mixed with a base and should never be applied directly to the skin in their pure form in case of an adverse allergic reaction.

An aromatherapist will 'design' an individual massage based on an accurate history taken from the patient and much experience in the use of essential oils. The oils will be chosen specifically to match the temperament of the patient and also to deal with any particular medical or emotional problems which may be troubling him or her.

Although there is no substitute for a long soothing

aromatherapy massage given by an expert, some of the techniques are not difficult to learn and massage can be used to great benefit at home using the following simple movements and suggestions.

Percussion (drumming or tapotement): Percussion is also called tapotement, which is derived from *tapoter,* a French word that means 'to drum' as of the fingers on a surface. As would be expected from its name, percussion is done with the edge of the hand with a quick chopping movement, although the strokes are not hard. This type of massage would be used on the back in places like the buttocks, waist and shoulders where there is a large expanse of muscular flesh.

Effleurage: Effleurage is the therapeutic movement used most often during a massage treatment and it consists of a simple, gentle stroking movement. Note that deep pressure should *never* be used by an untrained person. The strokes may be long or short, gentle or firm, but the whole hand should be used, always pushing the blood towards the heart, thus promoting venous return. This stroke promotes muscle relaxation and soothes the nerve endings.

Petrissage: In petrissage, the flesh is gently rolled between the thumbs and fingers in a movement not unlike kneading dough. This technique is best used on the back and on fatty areas. The idea is to stimulate the circulation and lymphatic flow and thereby increase the rate of toxin expulsion.

Head massage: Spread out the fingers and thumbs of both hands and with a little essential massage oil on the fingertips, place them on the scalp. Keep them in position and begin to move the scalp muscle over the bone by applying gentle pressure and circling slowly and firmly on the spot. Stop occasionally to move to a different area, then begin again, working gradually over the whole scalp.

Neck and shoulder massage: What follows can be used to relieve headaches, loosen shoulder muscles and provide a general feeling of relaxation. Neck and shoulder massage should be carried out with the patient sitting on a chair with some support in front. Place one hand at the base of the back of the neck and move it up to the hairline gently squeezing all the time. Return with a gentle downard stroke. Repeat several times.

Then starting at the bottom of the shoulder blades and using gentle effleurage movements, move your hands up each side of the spine to the base of the neck. Move your hands apart across the top of the shoulders and then bring them gently back down to the starting position. Repeat several times, finishing with a light return stroke.

Arm massage: Use effleurage and petrissage movements upwards in the direction of the armpit, concentrating on muscular and fleshy areas.

Back massage: Back massage helps to relax the whole body. The strokes should be carried out smoothly without lifting the hands from the back and using an appropriate essential oil. Applying thumb pressure to the channels on either side of the spine on the upper back will help respiratory problems. The same stroke on the lower back can relieve constipation and menstrual discomfort.

Avoiding the vertebrae, use gentle or firm effleurage movements. Begin by placing your hands, facing each other, on either side of the base of the spine. Move them up the back using your body weight to apply pressure. Stroke all the way from the lumbar to the shoulders, move the hands outwards across the shoulders and return slowly down the outer area of the back. Repeat this movement to induce deep relaxation.

To apply thumb pressure, place your hands at waist level with your thumbs in the hollows on either side of the spine and your fingers open and relaxed. Push your thumbs firmly up the channels for about 6 cm, relax them and then move them back about 2 cm. Continue in this way up to the neck. Then gently slide both hands back to the base of the spine. Repeat. Follow with with the first sequence.

Bathing

Most people have experienced the benefits of relaxing in a hot bath to which a proprietary perfumed preparation has been added. Most of these preparations contain essential oils used in aromatherapy. The addition of a number of drops of an essential oil to the bath water is soothing and relaxing, easing aches and pains, and can also have a stimulating effect, banishing tiredness and restoring energy. In addition, there is the added benefit of inhaling the vapours of the oil as they evaporate from the hot water.

Add a few drops (5–10) of essential oil to the bath water after the water has been drawn, then close the door to retain the aromatic vapours. The choice of oils is entirely up to the individual, depending on the desired effect, although those with sensitive skins are advised to have the oils ready diluted in a base oil prior to bathing.

Bathing in essential oils can stimulate and revive or relax and sedate depending on the oils selected: rosemary and pine can have a soothing effect on tired or aching limbs, chamomile and lavender are popular for relieving insomnia and anxiety, etc. A similar effect (although obviously not quite as relaxing) can be achieved whilst showering by soaking a wet sponge in essential oil mix, then rubbing it over the body under the warm spray.

Inhalation
Inhalation is thought to be the most direct and rapid means of treatment. This is because the molecules of the volatile essential oil act directly on the olfactory organs and are immediately perceived by the brain. A popular method is the time-honoured one of steam inhalation, in which a few drops of essential oil are added to hot water in a bowl. The person sits with his or her face above the mixture and covers the head, face and bowl with a towel so that the vapours do not escape. This can be repeated up to three times a day but should not be undertaken by people suffering from asthma.

Some essential oils can be applied directly to a handkerchief or onto a pillow and the vapours inhaled in this way.

Compresses
Compresses are effective in the treatment of a variety of muscular and rheumatic aches and pains as well as bruises and headaches. To prepare a compress, add 5 drops of oil to a small bowl of water. Soak a piece of flannel or other absorbent material in the solution. Squeeze out excess moisture (although the compress should remain fairly wet) and secure in position with a bandage or cling film.

For acute pain, the compress should be renewed when it has reached blood temperature, otherwise it should be left in position for a minimum of two hours and preferably overnight. Cold water should be used wherever fever or acute pain or hot swelling require treatment, whereas the water should be hot if the pain is chronic. If fever is present, the compress should be changed frequently.

How does it work?
Little is known about how essential oils actually affect the mind and the body, although research is currently ongoing in the USA and the UK. However, the effectiveness of aromatherapy has been supported by recent research in central Europe, the USA, the UK and Australia. It appears that most essential oils are antiseptic and bactericidal to some degree, whilst some even seem to be effective in fighting viral infections.

On inhalation, essential oil molecules are received by receptor cells in the lining of the nose, which will transmit signals to the brain. Electrochemical messages received by the olfactory centre in the brain then stimulate the release of powerful neurochemicals into the blood which will then be transported around the body. Molecules inhaled into the lungs may pass into the bloodstream and be disseminated in the same way.

When rubbed or massaged into the skin, essential oils will permeate the pores and hair follicles. From here, they can readily pass into the tiny blood vessels (known as capillaries) by virtue of their molecular structure, and then travel around the body. Once absorbed, the action of the oil depends upon its chemical constituents. Most essential oils are high in alcohols and esters, although a few contain a high concentration of phenols, aldehydes and ketones. The latter are powerful chemicals and their use should be avoided by all save the skilled professional.

Working with essential oils

Extraction: Since any part of a plant may produce essential oils, the method of extraction depends upon the site and accessibility of the essence in each particular case. In order to harvest the oils in appreciable amounts, it is usually necessary to collect a large quantity of the part of the plant needed and to subject the material to a process that releases the oil. One of the most common methods is *steam distillation*. Another method involves dissolving the plant material in a solvent, eg alcohol, and is called *solvent extraction*. A further method is called *maceration* in which the plant is soaked in hot oil. The plant cells collapse and release their essential oils, and the whole mixture is then separated and purified by a process called *defleurage*. If fat is used instead of oil, the process is called *enfleurage*. These methods produce a purer oil that is usually more expensive than one obtained by distillation. The essential oils used in aromatherapy tend to be costly as vast quantities of plant material are required to produce them and the methods used are complex and costly.

Storage and use of essential oils: Essential oils are highly concentrated, volatile and aromatic. They readily evaporate and change and deteriorate if exposed to light, heat and air. Hence pure oils need to be stored carefully in brown glass bottles at a moderate temperature away from direct light. They can be stored for one or two years in this way.

For most purposes in aromatherapy, essential oils are used in a dilute form, being added either to water or to another oil, called the *base* or *carrier*. The base is often a vegetable oil such as olive or safflower, which both have nutrient and beneficial properties. An essential/carrier oil mixture has a short useful life of two or three months and so they are usually mixed at the time of use and in small amounts.

Blending essential oils: Essences can be blended to treat specific ailments, and some aromatherapy books contain precise recipes for blends. When two or more essential oils are working together in harmony, this is known as a synergistic blend. Obviously, it takes many years of experience to know which combinations of plant essences will work most effectively together, but as a rough guide, oils extracted from plants of the same botanical family will usually blend and work well together, although it is by no means necessary to stick rigidly to this rule as other combinations may be just as successful.

A number of factors need to be taken into account when preparing a blend of oils for a patient, such as the nature of his/her complaint, his personality or frame of mind. For home use, it is not usually beneficial to blend more than three oils for any one preparation.

Base oils: Because essential oils are extremely concentrated and also because of their tendency to evaporate rapidly, they need to be diluted with carrier or base oils. Generally it is not advised that essential oils should be applied undiluted to the skin, although there are one or two specific exceptions. It is very important to use a high quality base oil, as oils such as baby or mineral oil have very poor penetrating qualities which will hamper the passage of the essential oil through the skin. Indeed, it would be better to use a good quality vegetable or nut oil for babies in preference to proprietary baby oils as the vegetable oil is more easily absorbed and contains more nutrients.

Although the choice of base oil is largely a matter of personal preference, it is useful to note that many vegetable oils possess therapeutic properties of their own. Any of sweet almond, soya bean, sunflower, jojoba, olive, grapeseed, hazelnut, avocado, corn or safflower oils will provide a suitable base for essential oils, although these should preferably be of the cold-pressed variety which have higher nutrient levels.

Pure essential oils should retain their potency for one to two years, but once diluted in a base oil will only last for three months or so before spoiling. They should also be stored at a fairly constant room temperature in corked dark glass bottles or flip-top containers as they will deteriorate quickly when subjected to extremes of light and temperature. Adding some vitamin E or wheatgerm oil to the mixture can help prolong its usefulness. For massage oils, it is best to make up a very small quantity of essential oil in base oil for each application because of its poor keeping qualities.

There is a very rough guide to the dilution of essential oils below. However, you will find many variations and differing opinions on this depending on the preference of individual therapists (and their recipes will differ accordingly).

Base oil	Essential oil
100ml	20–60 drops
25ml	7–25 drops
1 teaspoon (5ml)	3–5 drops

Some essential oils: The following section is by no means an exhaustive one, but aims to include some of the most popular oils readily available today. Similarly, while therapeutic uses have been suggested, therapists will differ in the choice of oils for particular complaints, just as a

GP may prescribe one remedy for a specific complaint, whereas his partner in the same practice may favour another treatment for the same complaint. While few, if any, are used specifically for the relief of back pain, many are helpful in promoting general well-being.

Basil (*Ociymum basilicum*)

Basil is now grown in many countries of the world although it originates from Africa. The herb has a long history of medicinal and culinary use, and was familiar to the Ancient Egyptian and Greek civilizations. Basil is sacred in the Hindu religion and has many medicinal uses in India and other Eastern countries. The whole plant is subjected to a process of steam distillation to obtain the essential oil used in aromatherapy. Basil is valued for its soothing and uplifting effects – its sweet, liquorice-like fragrance alleviates fatigue and depression and has a general tonic effect. Basil has a refreshing, invigorating effect and also has antiseptic properties. It can be effective in treating respiratory infections such as colds, bronchitis, asthma and sinusitis. It can also alleviate the symptoms of fever, gout and indigestion. It seems to be equally effective in relieving tired and over-worked muscles and is widely used in baths, inhalation and massage. Its strongly antiseptic effect sooths skin abrasions and assists the healing process. It also has insect repellent qualities. As a digestive aid, basil's antispasmodic effect has made it a favoured herb in cookery throughout the ages.

CAUTION: Basil should be avoided during pregnancy. It can also have a depressant effect, so it should be used in moderation. It is relatively non-toxic, but should be well diluted to avoid possible skin irritation.

Bergamot (*Citrus bergamia*)

Oil of bergamot is obtained from a plant that is a native species of some Asian and Eastern countries. The oil was first used and traded in Italy and derives its name from the northern city of Bergamo. In Italian medicine, it was popular as a remedy for feverish illnesses and to expel intestinal worms. It has also been used in cosmetics and perfumes, as the flavouring of Earl Grey tea, and in other foods. Recent research carried out in Italy indicates a wide variety of therapeutic applications for bergamot, including urinary tract and respiratory infections. Its strong antiseptic effect makes it a good choice for the treatment of skin, throat and mouth infections.

In particular, scalp and skin conditions such as psoriasis, acne and ulcers will often respond to treatment with bergamot, especially where stress and depression may have played a part in lowering resistance to infection. When combined with eucalyptus, its soothing effect will afford relief to sufferers of cold sores and shingles. Insomnia, anxiety and depression can be alleviated by the uplifting and refreshing nature of this oil. It also has a natural deodorizing effect and can be used both as a breath freshener and as a personal deodorant.

CAUTION: Bergamot can irritate the skin if used in concentrations in excess of 1%. It is phototoxic and should not be used in home-made suntan oil.

Chamomile, Roman (*Chamaemelum nobile*)

There are several varieties of chamomile, but Roman chamomile is the essential oil of choice for home use. It is used by therapists to treat many skin complaints and promotes the healing of burns, cuts, bites and inflammations. It is also effective in allergic conditions and can have a beneficial effect on menstrual problems when used regularly in the bath. It seems to be effective in reducing stress and anxiety and problems such as headache, migraine and insomnia. As an analgesic, it is used in the treatment of earache, toothache, neuralgia and abscesses, and it is popular for treating childhood illnesses.

CAUTION: Chamomile is generally non-toxic and non-irritant, but may cause dermatitis in very sensitive individuals.

Clary sage (*Salvia sclarea*)

Clary sage is possessed of antispasmodic, antidepressant, balsamic, carminative, tonic, aperitive, astringent, anti-inflammatory, bactericidal and antiseptic qualities. It is valuable in stress-related conditions and has an antihypertensive effect. A thick mucilage, which was traditionally used for removing particles of dust from the eyes, can be made from the seeds. Clary sage is also indicated in the treatment of colds and throat infections, and for regulating menstrual problems and soothing problem skin, particularly if dry or sensitive.

CAUTION: Clary sage should be avoided during pregnancy and also not used in conjunction with alcohol consumption. However, in general, clary sage has very low toxicity levels and is therefore preferable to garden sage for use in aromatherapy.

Eucalyptus (*Eucalyptus globulus*)

Eucalyptus is a native species of Australia and Tasmania but it is now grown in many countries throughout the world. The plant has a characteristic pungent odour, and the oil obtained from it has disinfectant and antiseptic properties, clears the nasal passages and acts as a painkiller. The leaves and twigs are subjected to a process of steam distillation in order to obtain the essential oil used in aromatherapy. The diluted oil is used for muscular and rheumatic aches and pains, skin disorders, such as ringworm, insect bites, headaches and neuralgia, shingles, respiratory and bronchitic infections and fevers. Eucalyptus is used in many household products and in remedies for coughs and colds. Its analgesic properties are often used to ease the discomfort of shingles, chickenpox and herpes as well as to soothe muscular aches and sprains.

CAUTION: When diluted, eucalyptus oil is safe to use externally, but it can be fatal if taken internally.

Geranium (*Pelargonium graveolens*)

Geranium is an excellent 'all-round' oil, with a wide range of uses, particularly for menopausal problems and premenstrual tension. Its diuretic quality makes it a wise choice for fluid retention, and cellulitis and mastitis often respond well to it. For skin conditions and emotional disorders, it is a popular choice in the bath and in massage oil. Serious skin conditions often respond to its antiseptic and antifungal qualities.

CAUTION: Generally a non-toxic and non-irritant oil, geranium oil may cause contact dermatitis in hypersensitive individuals.

Jasmine (*Jasminum officinalis*)

Because jasmine is so costly, it is not much used in home aromatherapy, but like all essential oils it does have therapeutic uses. Its heady, uplifting scent makes it useful in the treatment of stress-related illnesses. It also has a smoothing effect on skin and is a valuable component in skin-care preparations. It also seems to have a regulating effect on the menstrual cycle, and has been successfully used for throat problems, coughs and catarrh. However, as there are many less expensive oils that will perform these functions, jasmine's main use is as a fragrance ingredient in perfumes.

CAUTION: Although a non-toxic and non-irritant oil, jasmine oil has, on occasion, caused an allergic reaction.

Lavender (*Lavendula vera*)

The highly perfumed lavender is a native species of the Mediterranean but has long been popular as a garden plant in Britain and many other countries. It has antiseptic, tonic and relaxing properties, and the essential oil used in aromatherapy is obtained by subjecting the flowers to a process of steam distillation.

It is considered to be one of the safest preparations and is used in the treatment of a wide range of disorders.

Lavender is an appetite stimulant, a tonic and an antispasmodic. It is particularly effective in the treatment of minor burns and scalds, wounds, sores and varicose ulcers, and is generally one of the most versatile and widely used oils for healing. It also has a strong antiseptic effect and is employed in many cosmetic preparations and as an insect repellent. It is also used in the treatment of muscular aches and pains, respiratory problems, influenza, digestive problems and genito-urinary problems such as cystitis and dysmenorrhoea. Its soothing effect is recommended for headaches and premenstrual tension. Lavender is a very safe oil and can even be applied undiluted to the skin.

Marjoram, Sweet (*Origanum marjorana*)

Marjoram can be extremely effective in reducing the pain and swelling of muscular damage, bruises and sprains, and arthritis. It has an extremely hypnotic effect, which is useful in inducing sleep and calming emotions, especially when used in the bath. It can also be effective in menstrual problems. Marjoram is also a popular treatment for colds and coughs, bronchitis and asthma, and has a carminative and antispasmodic action on colic, constipation and flatulence.

CAUTION: Marjoram should be avoided by pregnant women as it has a strong emmenagogic effect.

Neroli (*Citrus aurantium*)

Neroli is an extremely expensive oil to produce because of the volume of flowers required, but it is very much in demand because of its wonderful aroma. This is frequently harnessed in massage oil because of its power to uplift, calm and relax. It is also believed to have qualities that are beneficial to the skin, and is widely used to prevent stretch marks and scarring, to reduce thread veins and as an aid for dry, sensitive skin. Neroli's stress-relieving qualities indicate its use in a wide variety of complaints, ranging from colitis and diarrhoea to palpitations, insomnia and premenstrual tension.

Patchouli (*Pogostemon patchouli*)

Patchouli possesses a soothing, calming earthy scent. It is a good antiseptic with anti-inflammatory properties, which makes it a sensible choice in the treatment of minor burns. Patchouli has also been credited with aphrodisiac powers, and is excellent for relieving a variety of skin disorders including acne, athlete's foot, eczema and dry and cracked skin. It is also used for treating poisonous snakebites in Japan and Malaysia.

Petitgrain (*Citrus bigordia*)

Petitgrain can be used as a mild antidepressant substitute for neroli, and is effective in the alleviation of anxiety and insomnia. It is also valuable in skincare, having a balancing and toning effect on greasy skin conditions. In the digestive system, it reduces the symptoms of dyspepsia and flatulence.

Pine (*Pinus sylvestris*)

Pine has a strong antiseptic quality, valued for its effectiveness in treating respiratory conditions and in relieving asthma, blocked sinuses and catarrh when used as an inhalation. Its stimulating effect also makes it a good choice as a warming massage oil for muscular pains and strains. It has a multitude of other applications for cuts and sores, arthritis and rheumatism, cystitis and urinary tract infections, fatigue, stress, anxiety and neuralgia.

CAUTION: Those with a tendency towards sensitive skin should avoid bathing in pine oil. Pine oil should only be used under the direction of a trained aromatherapist and is unsafe for home use.

Rose (*Rosa centifola*)

Rose has a supremely feminine and deeply sensual aroma, which is the traditional mainstay of the perfume industry. Rose oil has a wonderful antidepressant effect that may be harnessed in body and face massages, baths or vaporizers to treat anxiety, stress and depression. It also has a gentle balancing effect on gynaecological disorders and is said to have aphrodisiac properties.

Rosemary (*Rosemarinus officinalis*)

Rosemary has a wide application and is effective in the treatment of numerous complaints. Possessing a powerful aroma, rosemary is favoured as a decongestant in inhalation and an invigorating muscle-strengthening massage oil. Skin and hair problems can respond well to rosemary, and gargling with it will freshen the breath. Above all, rosemary seems to possess remarkable memory and concentration-enhancing properties. Other therapeutic uses are in digestive disorders, headaches and stress.

CAUTION: Rosemary oil should be avoided during pregnancy and should not be used by epileptics.

Sandalwood (*Santalum album*)
Its preservative powers are often employed to lengthen the life of creams and potions. Sandalwood is a wonderful facial oil, with a soothing emollient effect on dry or sensitive skin. This oil also has a powerful relaxing effect and can alleviate upset stomachs, especially where nervous tension or stress has been a causative factor. Sandalwood also seems to have a powerful antiseptic effect that is particularly useful in the treatment of cystitis and urinary tract infections. It is also favoured for menstrual problems, for catarrh and as a sedative.

Ylang Ylang (*Cananga odorata*)
Ylang ylang is a native species of the Far Eastern islands of Indonesia, the Philippines, Java and Madagascar. To obtain the essential oil used in aromatherapy, the flowers are subjected to a process of steam distillation.Like most essential oils ylang ylang has a strong antiseptic effect, but it is best known for its euphoric and aphrodisiac properties. The nervous

system can also benefit greatly from its relaxing powers, and its antidepressant powers can also be harnessed to treat mild shock, anger and stress. It has a calming effect on the heartbeat rate and can be used to relieve palpitations, tachycardia, hypertension (raised blood pressure), depression and shock. It is used widely as an ingredient in skincare products, having a wonderful tonic effect and gentle action.

CAUTION: Ylang Ylang oil is generally very safe, although sensitization has been reported in a small number of cases. Used excessively, it can cause nausea or headache.

Hydrotherapy

Introduction

Hydrotherapy is the use of water to heal and ease a variety of ailments, and the water may be used in a number of different ways. The healing properties of water have been recognized since ancient times, notably by the Greek, Roman and Turkish civilizations but also by people in Europe and China. Most people know the benefits of a hot bath in relaxing the body, relieving muscular aches and stiffness, and helping to bring about restful sleep. Hot water or steam causes blood vessels to dilate, opens skin pores and stimulates perspiration, and relaxes limbs and muscles. A cold bath or shower acts in the opposite way and is refreshing and invigorating. The cold causes blood vessels in the skin to constrict and blood is diverted to internal tissues and organs to maintain the core temperature of the body. Applications of cold water or ice reduce swelling and bruising and cause skin pores to close.

In orthodox medicine, hydrotherapy is used as a technique of physiotherapy for people recovering from serious injuries with problems of muscle wastage. Also, it is used for people with joint problems and those with severe physical disabilities. Many hospitals also offer the choice of a water birth to expectant mothers, and this has become an increasingly popular method of childbirth. Hydrotherapy may be offered as a form of treatment for other medical conditions in *naturopathy,* using the techniques listed below. It is wise to obtain medical advice before proceeding with hydrotherapy, and this is especially important for elderly persons, children and those with serious conditions or illnesses.

Treatment
Hot baths: Hot baths are used to ease muscle and joint pains and inflammation. Also, warm or hot baths, with the addition of various substances, such as seaweed extract, to the water, may be used to help the healing of some skin conditions or minor wounds. After childbirth, frequent bathing in warm water to which a mild antiseptic has been added is recommended to heal skin tears.

Most people know the relaxing benefits of a hot bath. A bath with the temperature between 36.5°C and 40°C (98°F and 104°F) is very useful as a means of muscle relaxation. To begin with, 5 minutes immersion in a bath of this temperature is enough. This can be stepped up to 10 minutes a day, as long as no feelings of weakness or dizziness arise. It is important to realize that a brief hot bath has quite a different effect from a long one.

There is nothing to be gained by prolonging a hot bath in the hope of increasing the benefit. Immersion in hot water acts not only on the surface nerves but also on the autonomic nervous system (which is normally outside our control), as well as the hormone-producing glands, particularly the adrenals, which become less active. A hot bath is sedative, but a hot bath that is prolonged into a long soak has quite the opposite effect.

Cold baths: Cold baths are used to improve blood flow to internal tissues and organs and to reduce swellings. The person may sit for a moment in shallow cold water with additional water being splashed onto exposed skin. An inflamed, painful part may be immersed in cold water to reduce swelling. The person is not allowed to become chilled, and this form of treatment is best suited for those able to dry themselves rapidly with a warm towel. It is not advisable for people with serious conditions or for the elderly or very young.

Neutral baths: There are many nerve endings on the skin surface and these deal with the reception of stimuli. More of these are cold receptors than heat receptors. If water of a different temperature to that of the skin is applied, it will either conduct heat to it or absorb heat from it. These stimuli have an influence on the sympathetic nervous system and can affect the hormonal system. The greater the difference between the temperature of the skin and the water applied, the greater will be the potential for physiological reaction. Conversely, water that is the same temperature as the body has a marked relaxing and sedative effect on the nervous system. This is of value in states of stress, and has led to the development of the so-called 'neutral bath'.

Before the development of tranquillizers, the most dependable and effective method of calming an agitated patient was the use of a neutral bath. The patient was placed in a tub of water, the temperature of which was maintained at between 33.5°C and 35.6°C (92°F to 96°F) often for over 3 hours, and sometimes for as long as 24 hours. Obviously, this is not a practical proposition for the average tense person.

As a self-help measure, the neutral bath does, however, offer a means of sedating the nervous system if used for relatively short periods. It is important to maintain the water temperature at the above level, and for this a bath thermometer should be used. The bathroom itself should be kept warm to prevent any chill in the air.

Half an hour of immersion in a bath like this will have a sedative, or even soporific, effect. It places no strain on the heart, circulation or nervous system, and achieves muscular relaxation as well as a relaxation and expansion of the blood vessels: all of these promote relaxation. This bath can be used in conjunction with other methods of relaxation, such as breathing techniques and meditation, to make it an even more efficient way of coping with stress. It can be used daily if necessary.

Steam baths: Steam baths, along with saunas and Turkish baths, are used to encourage sweating and the opening of skin pores and have a cleansing and refreshing effect. The body may be able to eliminate harmful substances in this way and treatment finishes with a cool bath.

Sitz baths: Sitz baths are usually given as a treatment for painful conditions with broken skin, such as piles or anal fissure, and also for ailments affecting the urinary and genital organs. The person sits in a specially designed bath that has two compartments, one with warm water, the other with cold. First, the person sits in the warm water, which covers the lower abdomen and hips, with the feet in the cold water compartment. After three minutes, the patient changes round and sits in the cold water with the feet in the warm compartment.

Hot and cold sprays: Hot and cold sprays of water may be given for a number of different disorders but are not recommended for those with serious illnesses, elderly people or young children.

Wrapping: Wrapping is used for feverish conditions, backache and bronchitis. A cold wet sheet that has been squeezed out is wrapped around the person, followed by a dry sheet and warm blanket. These are left in place until the inner sheet has dried and the coverings are then removed. The body is sponged with tepid water (at blood heat) before being dried with a towel. Sometimes the wrap is applied to a smaller area of the body, such as the lower abdomen, to ease a particular problem, usually constipation.

Cold packs: The description that follows was a treatment used in the past but seldom if ever nowadays when we associate cold packs with the frozen gel packs that are used to treat areas of pain and inflammation.

Historically cold packs were described by the famous 19th-century Bavarian pastor, Sebastian Kniepp, in his famous treatise *My Water Cure*, in which he explained the advantages of hydrotherapy. A cold pack was really a warm pack – the name comes from the cold nature of the initial application. For a cold pack you needed: a large piece of cotton material; a large piece of flannel or woollen (blanket) material; a rubber sheet to protect the bed; safety pins and a hot water bottle.

First, the cotton material was soaked in very cold water, wrung out well and placed on the flannel material that was spread out on the rubber sheet on the bed. The person who was having the treatment lay on top of the damp cotton material, which was then folded round his trunk and he was then covered up at once with the flannel material which was safety-pinned firmly in place.

The top bed covers were pulled up and a hot water bottle provided. The initial cold application produced a reaction that drew fresh blood to the surface of the body; this warmth, being well insulated, was retained by the damp material. The cold pack turned into a warm pack, which gradually, over a period of 6 to 8 hours, baked itself dry. Usually lots of sweat was produced, so it was necessary to wash the materials well before using again.

The pack could be slept in – in fact it was said to encourage deeper, more refreshing sleep. Larger, whole body packs were also used, which covered not only the trunk but extend from the armpits to the feet, encasing the recipient in a cocoon of warmth.

Flotation: A form of sensory deprivation, flotation involves lying face up in an enclosed, dark tank of warm, heavily salted water. There is no sound, except perhaps some natural music to bring the client into a dreamlike state. It is exceptionally refreshing and induces a deep, relaxing sleep.

16. Conclusion

In conclusion, it is hoped that whether a sufferer or not, the reader will find after reading this guide to back pain that he or she is better-informed and will have gained some understanding of how best to deal with back pain, should the need arise.